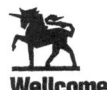

Mit
freundlichen
Empfehlungen

**Wellcome
GmbH**

P. Berlit P. M. Moore (Eds.)

Vasculitis, Rheumatic Disease and the Nervous System

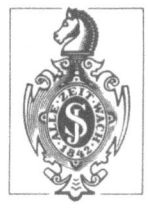

Springer-Verlag
Berlin Heidelberg GmbH

Peter Berlit, Prof. Dr. med.
Neurologische Klinik mit klinischer Neurophysiologie
Alfried Krupp Krankenhaus Essen
Alfried-Krupp-Straße 21
D-4300 Essen 1, Germany

Patricia M. Moore, M.D. Associate Professor
Wayne State University
Department of Neurology
6E University Health Center
4201 St. Antoine, Detroit, Michigan 48208
USA

ISBN 978-3-540-54853-9   ISBN 978-3-642-77122-4 (eBook)
DOI 10.1007/978-3-642-77122-4

25/3145/5 4 3 2 1 0 – Printed on acid-free paper

Contents

Contributors

Arlt Andreas C.
Klinische Rheumatologie, Ratzeburger Allee 160, 2400 Lübeck 1, FRG

Berlit Peter
Neurologische Klinik mit Klinischer Neurophysiologie, Alfried Krupp von Bohlen
und Halbach Krankenhaus, Alfried Krupp Straße 21, 4300 Essen, FRG

Bluestein Harry G.
Division of Rheumatology, Department of Medicine, University of California, San
Diego, 225 Dickinson Street, San Diego, California 92103, USA

Gretz Norbert
Nephrologische Klinik, Klinikum Mannheim, 6800 Mannheim 1, FRG

Gross Wolfgang L.
Klinische Rheumatologie, Ratzeburger Allee 160, 2400 Lübeck 1, FRG

Moore Patricia M.
Department of Neurology, 6E University Health Center, 4201 St. Antoine, Detroit,
Michigan 48201, USA

Peter Hans H.
Abteilung für Rheumatologie und Klinische Immunologie,
Medizinische Universitätsklinik, Hugstetterstr. 55, 7800 Freiburg, FRG

Schmitt Wilhelm H.
Klinische Rheumatologie, Ratzeburger Allee 160, 2400 Lübeck 1, FRG

Schwartz Andreas
Neurologische Klinik, Klinikum Mannheim, Universität Heidelberg, 6800 Mannheim,
FRG

Storch-Hagenlocher Brigitte
Neurologische Klinik, Universität Heidelberg, Im Neuenheimer Feld 400,
6900 Heidelberg, FRG

Täschner Karl-Ludwig
Psychiatrische Klinik, Bürgerhospital, Tunzhofer Str. 14–16, 7000 Stuttgart 1, FRG

Immunologic Diagnosis of Vasculitis

Hans H. Peter

Introduction

A variety of immunopathologic mechanisms are involved in the etiopatho-genesis of vasculitis [1, 8]. Besides infectious agents and their immunologic footprints, notably autoimmune diseases, malignancies, and toxic-allergic reactions have to be considered as possible underlying causes. Numerous attempts have been undertaken to classify vasculitides, but so far none has been satisfactory [6]. A still widely accepted scheme distinguishes *primary and secondary vasculitides,* although new classifications according to immu-nologic parameters (e.g., antinuclear antibody, ANA-, or antineutrophilic cytoplasmic autoantibody, ANCA-positive, hyper-, hypo-, or normocomple-mentemic vasculitis) may soon prevail. Table 1 summarizes the most fre-quent vasculitis syndromes and some of the associated key laboratory find-ings. In Table 2 an attempt is made to group vasculitides into ANCA positive, ANA positive and ANCA/ANA negative ones.

2 The Clinical Approach

Any clinical suspicion of vasculitis requires a thorough medical history to be taken, including family and personal history, habits, and occupation (Table 3). Subsequently a careful *physical examination* followed by a *diagnostic screening program* as shown in Table 4 are mandatory. The listed tests should not be performed rigidly but rather adapted to the individual needs of each patient. Diagnostic hallmarks in vasculitis are a variety of bacterial, viral, autoantigen, and drug-related antibodies. Furthermore, circulating immune complexes, complement split products (C3a, C3d), and acute phase proteins (C-reactive protein, fibrinogen, ferritin, haptoglobin, C3), as well as paraproteins, cryoglobulin, and cryofibrinogen have to be considered.

3 The Immunologic Approach

The clinical manifestations of vasculitis depend on the type of antigen involved (autoantigen, foreign antigen), the predominant immunopatho-

P. Berlit, P. M. Moore (Eds.)
Vasculitis, Rheumatic Disease
and the Nervous System
© Springer-Verlag Berlin Heidelberg 1993

The classic reaction was produced by active immunization of an experimental animal with heterologous albumin (resulting in specific antibody formation), followed by intradermal or subcutaneous injection of the same antigen. Histologic lesions are evident 4–10 h after injection of the antigen into a sensitized animal. Extensive studies have examined the characteristics of complexes required to produce skin reactivity. Larger-sized lattices are more effective in activating complement and mediating pathologic effects. The antibody type and subclass also determine subsequent tissue damage. Histopathologic features are well described. The local lesions are characterized by increased vascular permeability, edema, and polymorphonuclear leukocyte (PMN) infiltration of the postcapillary venules, followed by hemorrhagic necrosis. Immune complexes can be identified by immunofluorescence early but are usually removed by neutrophils within 24–48 h. Subsequent activation of complement initiates immune adherence reactions, including release of chemotactic factors and anaphylatoxins (C3a and C5) and formation of the membrane attack complex. Infiltrating neutrophils bind to the complexes. There is phagocytosis and release of inflammatory peptides and oxygen radicals. The generation of both peroxide and hydroxyl radicals appears important in mediating injury. Iron may potentiate the damage. Infiltration of the vessels with mononuclear cells and plasma cells occurs later.

Systemic immune complex disease may be acute or chronic, depending on the amount of antigen, the route of administration, and host factors such as antibody response and integrity of the reticuloendothelial system (RES). Acute serum sickness is the model for circulating immune complex vascular disease. Antibodies react with free antigens to form circulating complexes.

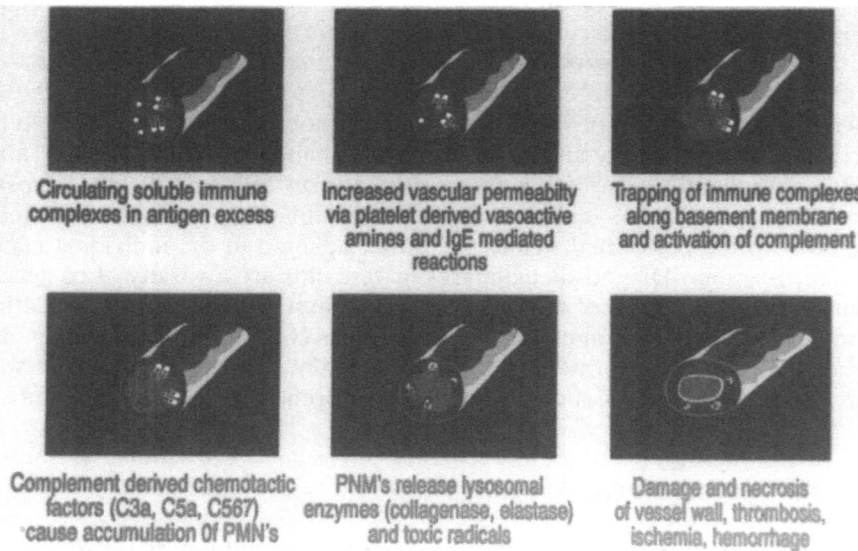

Fig. 1. Immune complex-mediated vasculitis

Under normal circumstances these are removed by the RES and cause no damage. In some situations the capacity for removal of these complexes is exceeded and, if additional conditions are also appropriate, the complexes may be deposited in the blood vessels. The immune complexes most likely to produce vascular disease are large and of high valence. Among the factors which determine the localization of the immune complex deposits are hemodynamic forces and charges in the vessel wall. Conditions conducive to intravascular deposition of complexes and subsequent inflammation are:

1. Increased vascular permeability with filtration of immune complexes by the elastic lamina of arteries or the basement membrane of venules, this is usually initiated by immunoglobulin E (IgE) and mediated by vasoactive amines
2. Soluble large latticed complexes (containing more than 2 antibody molecules or $>Ag_2Ab_2$), formed under conditions of slight antigen excess.

The trapped immune complexes activate complement, leading to an influx of PMNs and, later, macrophages. The PMNs release proteolytic enzymes and toxic radicals which destroy the functional and physical integrity of the vessel wall. Thrombosis, occlusion, and hemorrhage ensue. Lesions usually heal with prominent scarring.

Deposition of immune complexes also varies with the type of vasculature. Renal glomeruli and the choroid plexus have fenestrated endothelia which readily filter, or trap, large molecules [14]. During experimental immune complex disease, antigen–antibody complexes are detectable in the glomeruli long after they have been cleared from other vessels. In the glomeruli, immune complexes coalesce into larger immune deposits which may then lead to further deposition of complexes and even larger lattices. This phenomenon may be exacerbated by the fixed negative charge of the basement membrane [2, 7]. These observations offer an explanation of why renal disease is prominent even when other organs are spared. Similarly amplified immune complex deposition may well occur in the choroid plexus, but the clinical effects of this are difficult to determine. Immunoglobulins and immune complexes are present in the choroid plexus of rabbits with acute serum sickness and humans with systemic lupus erythematosus, but the effects are unclear. Experimental models indicate altered behavior in animals, but immunoglobulin binding to the choroid plexus is found in patients both with and without neurologic abnormalities.

Chronic immune complex disease resulting from repeated exposure to smaller doses of antigen differs from acute immune complex disease. Typically, rabbits develop glomerulonephritis but not arteritis. Administration of split doses of antigen to rabbits who are high antibody producers may, however, result in extraglomerular vascular disease. In other animal models the vascular injury also depends on the host's antibody response. Mice that produce low titers of antibodies in response to antigen demonstrate a degenerative vasculopathy associated with the deposition of immune complexes in the vessel wall. Mice that produce higher levels of antibody show a more prominent inflammatory response. This may well be similar to systemic lupus erythematosus in humans: in association with chronically low levels of circulating immune complexes a degenerative vasculopathy occurs, but only rarely is a vasculitis in the CNS present.

2.2 Direct Antibody-Mediated Changes

The occurrence of blood vessel-specific antibody-mediated vasculitis remains conjectural although recent studies support such a mechanism in Kawasaki's syndrome [13]. Kawasaki's syndrome is an acute childhood illness characterized histologically by a panvasculitis with endothelial cell necrosis, immunoglobulin deposition, and infiltration of monocuclear cells into small and medium-sized blood vessels. Sera from patients with Kawasaki's syndrome contain IgM and IgG antibodies cytotoxic for cultured endothelial cells which have been stimulated with γ-interferon, interleukin 1 (IL-1), or tumor necrosis factor (TNF) [13]; these antibodies have no effect on endothelial cells that have not been stimulated. All of these cytokines induce class II MHC and adhesion molecules on endothelial cells as well as stimulating the endothelial cells to release their own cytokines. In Kawasaki's syndrome, demonstrably high levels of circulating IL-1 and TNF are required for the endothelial cell damage.

Another autoantibody with strong associations with a systemic vasculitis is the cANCA (classic antineutrophilic cytoplasmic antibody) present in patients with Wegener's granulomatosis [20]. The antineutrophilic cytoplasmic antibodies react with constituents of neutrophil primary granules and monocyte lysosmes. The target of cANCA appears to be proteinase 3. Although potential mechanisms for in vitro changes in endothelial cells secondary to antibody to a cytoplasmic white blood cell antigen exist, there is as yet no evidence that in vivo this antibody causes a vasculitis.

2.3 Cell-Mediated Changes

Recent studies on the role of the endothelial cell as an antigen-presenting cell (APC) support the theory that many of the vasculitic syndromes result from local immune reactions rather than from circulating factors or complexes (Fig. 2). Histologic studies sustain this; in these vasculitides infiltrates are composed primarily of lymphocytes and macrophages with few, if any, neutrophils. There is no deposition of immunoglobulins or complement. Unique features of endothelial cells and T cells mark them as the most likely participants in the cell-mediated vasculitides.

Endothelial cells are in an immunologically unique position: their membrane proteins are continuously exposed to lymphocytes; they can function as antigen-presenting cells, and they secrete cytokines. Endothelial

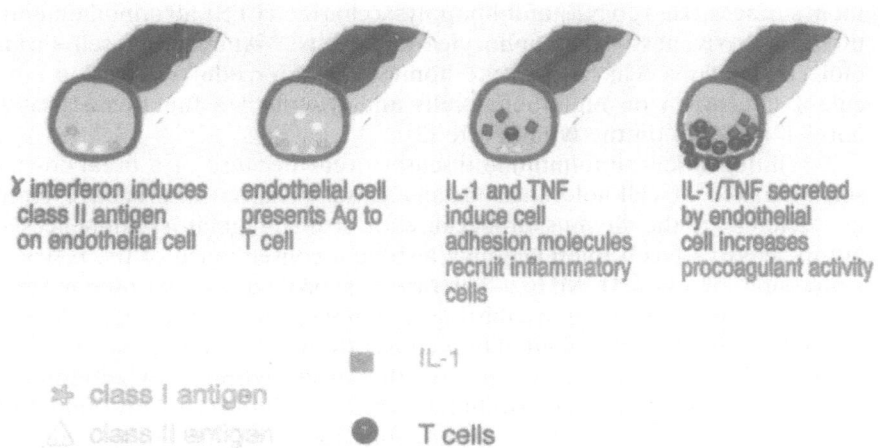

γ interferon induces class II antigen on endothelial cell

endothelial cell presents Ag to T cell

IL-1 and TNF induce cell adhesion molecules recruit inflammatory cells

IL-1/TNF secreted by endothelial cell increases procoagulant activity

■ IL-1

⇶ class I antigen

△ class II antigen

● T cells

Fig. 2. Potential mechanisms of mononuclear cell-associated vasculitis.

cells present antigens and may present them in diseases as diverse as allogenic transplantation reactions, viral CNS infections, and multiple sclerosis. Endothelial cells can express MHC antigens and can be induced to express Fc and complement receptors. Class II molecules on endothelial cells can both be induced by T cells (by γ-interferon) and can induce T-cell proliferation. With class II molecules endothelial cells present antigen to T helper cells. The T cells then recruit the appropriate immune response via cytokines [5].

Alternatively, the endothelial cells may be perceived by the T cells as foreign or altered, as may occur in a viral infection. The endothelial cells themselves are then the target of cytotoxic T cells. Lymphocytes, after immune stimulation in mixed lymphocyte culture, stimulate angiogenesis in vivo and endothelial cell proliferation in vivo. IL-1 can be synthesized by the endothelial cell, a process which appears to be induced by TNF [4].

Additionally and perhaps centrally in some vasculitides, the endothelium releases mediators which govern chemotaxis and adherence of leukocytes, changes in permeability of the vessel wall, and molecular and cellular transport across the endothelial barrier [11]. Cytokines such as interferon, IL-1, and TNF released during the inflammatory response increase class II expression by the endothelial cells, thereby recruiting more inflammatory cells. IL-1 and other cytokines also induce thromboplastin, prostacyclin, and platelet activating factors from endothelial cells, which results in altered vascular permeability and thrombosis [12].

Endothelial cells also direct the traffic of circulating lymphocytes. Organ-specific homing of lymphocytes occurs by interactions of lymphocytes and endothelial cells [8, 19]. Endothelial cells effect adhesion of lymphocytes to

their surfaces. IL-1, TNF, and lipopolysaccharide (LPS) all stimulate endothelial adhesiveness for lymphocytes and PMNs. Among the cell surface
molecules involved in lymphocyte homing are intercellular adhesion molecule 1 (ICAM-1) on endothelial cells and lymphocyte function-associated
antigen (LFA-1) on the lymphocyte [3].

T cell-dependent autoimmune diseases occur because of a breakdown in
self-tolerance. T-cell tolerance usually exists because autoreactive clones
are deleted in the thymus or because of strong regulatory influences on
autoreactivity. T-cell tolerance may also be a consequence of the restricted
expression of class II MHC. Tolerance is broken as a consequence of
aberrant expression, thus permitting a response by CD4 T cells. Whether
the initial stimulus for inflammation comes from the T cell or the endothelial cell probably varies depending on the specific disease or condition. T
cells may provide the signal/stimulus (such as γ-interferon) to endothelial
cells to express class II, which subsequently recruits T cells to the site. This
mutual stimulatory interaction is likely responsible for a prompt immunologic response to tissue injury [8]. It may also provide conditions for
autoimmune disease. Alternatively, T cells may respond to specific neoantigens on endothelial cells. Rather than a breakdown in self-tolerance
this may explain frequently encountered phenomena such as perivascular
cuffing; this process may also occur in diseases such as CNS vasculitis
[10, 16].

Why are certain idiopathic and known secondary vasculitides restricted
to the CNS? The answer is not known and remains the center of current
investigation. Arteries of the CNS possess both antigens, enzymes, and
structural features which distinguish them from arteries of other tissue.
Evidence that CNS arteries have unique enzymes and phenotypic markers
has accumulated over the past few years. Most of the studies have centered
on the endothelial cell. Brain microvascular endothelial cells appear to
have alkaline phosphatase, gamma-glutamyl transpeptidase activity, and
brain-associated Thy-1 (BAT-1) not present in endothelial cells from other
organs.

2.4 Other Mechanisms

Although most current research in cell-mediated vasculitis is centered on the
endothelial cell, recent evidence suggests that particularly in the nervous
system, other cells may be the primary antigen-presenting cells. Information
from chimeric animals shows that perivascular microglial cells present antigen [9]. Other investigators think that the smooth muscle cells in the vessel
wall are potential initiators of vascular inflammation [6]. It remains difficult
to localize the inciting cells in human neurologic vascular diseases from
current in vitro or experimental animal studies in vivo. These studies do,
however, enable us to ask more specific questions in histologic samples from
patients and to explore new therapies.

2.4.1 Granulomatous

The presence of giant cells and granulomas in certain vasculitides suggests that macrophages and monocytes may be involved but their roles are not well delineated. Granulomata result from several pathways in the cell-mediated and the immune complex-mediated inflammation. Granulomas are a central part of the infiltrate in certain diseases such as Wegener's granulomatosis, tuberculosis, and sarcoidosis and a variable feature in other diseases. As mentioned above, because numerous, usually unknown, antigens may incite the initial reaction, it remains difficult to predict when granulomas will dominate the infiltrate.

2.4.2 Eosinophilic

A role for eosinophils in certain vasculitides is postulated. The Churg-Strauss syndrome is characterized by eosinophilia and a granulomatous vasculitis. Biopsy specimens from a patient with Churg-Strauss angiitis revealed a large amount of eosinophilic cationic protein and eosinophilic protein X in the granulomas. The role of eosinophils in inflammatory reactions and tissue injury continues to be investigated [12]. Eosinophils secrete inflammatory lipid mediators, including prostaglandins. Eosinophilic major basic protein appears to be toxic to, at least, bronchial epithelium. In addition, eosinophils can be stimulated to be adherent to cultured endothelial cells. The stimulus and mechanisms for in vivo vascular damage-associated eosinophilic infiltration has not yet been determined.

3 Inflammation Secondary to Vessel Injury

Vascular inflammation may also occur in areas of vascular injury. Possible cellular events include primary platelet adhesion with a secondary release of inflammatory mediators; this may be the cause of vessel inflammation in atherosclerosis and malignant hypertension. Damaged vessels may also expose antigens previously hidden from immune recognition; these "neoantigens" may then be the target of either antibody- or cell-mediated immune reactions.

4 Animal Experimental Models

There are a number of species of vertebrates that develop diseases in which vascular inflammation is a major component of the clinical illness (Table 1). Several of these diseases are well studied and provide information on the variety of mechanisms producing vasculitis and the temporal course of histologic changes.

Table 1. Animal diseases with vascular inflammation as a major component

Animal model	Etiology	Mechanism
Aleutian mink disease	Virus	Immune complex
Equine viral arteritis	Virus	Cell mediated
Mycoplasma infection of turkeys	*Mycoplasma*	Toxic
MRL/*lpr* mice	Genetic	Immune complex
Toxic vasculitis of monkey	Drugs: amphetamine	?

Aleutian mink disease is a naturally occurring disease caused by a viral infection of genetically susceptible mink. Circulating infectious virus–antibody complexes deposit in the blood vessels. Clinically, the animals develop progressive weight loss, splenomegaly, lymphadenopathy, hepatomegaly, glomerulonephritis, widespread plasma cell infiltration, and necrotizing arteritis. Histologically, a segmental polymorphonuclear infiltrate predominates. IgG, C3, and virus can be detected in the intima and media of affected vessels. Fibrinoid necrosis (granular, eosinophilic hyaline-appearing material) subsequently appears. Various stages of lesions are present in different arteries. Lesions heal incompletely and fibrosis is frequent [18].

Another naturally occurring virus is pathogenic for vascular inflammation. Equine viral arteritis, clinically characterized by rapid-onset fever, leukopenia, and edema, results from a viral infection of the vascular endothelium. Endothelial swelling is followed by a mononuclear cell infiltrate, thinned vessel walls, and a leaky basement membrane. Viral antigen but no antibody is detectable in the endothelium by immunfluorescence. The lesions characteristically heal with little or no scarring.

A neurologically specific vasculitis occurs in *Mycoplasma gallisepticum* infection of turkeys. Inoculation of turkeys with viable *Mycoplasma gallisepticum* results in rapid onset of arteritic lesions. The mechanism appears to be toxic. Viable organisms are necessary to produce the disease, which can be treated with antibiotics but not corticosteroids.

Several strains of inbred mice develop arteritis. The etiology is unknown and there is no evidence for an infectious cause. These animals do have circulating autoantibodies. MRL/*lpr* mice develop prominent autoantibody formation and histopathologic changes similar to some human collagen vascular diseases. There is no evidence for an infectious etiology. Some of these animals develop a systemic vasculitis which appears to be accelerated by the lpr gene. In other studies the pathogenesis of vascular pathology appears to be related to the levels of circulating autoantibodies to which the animals are exposed. Animals with high levels of autoantibodies are more prone to develop a inflammatory vascular disease, while animals with low levels of circulating antibodies develop a degenerative vasculopathy without evidence of inflammation. In these animals the type of infiltrate provides information on the pathogenesis. Infiltration with neutrophils is associated with immune complex deposition, while a predominantly mononuclear cell infiltrate is much less likely associated with antibody or immune complex deposition [17].

5 Conclusion

In conclusion, the study of the interactions between the vessel wall and immune cells in health and disease continues to be productive for both the clinician and the scientist. Our information is expanding rapidly, and it is to be hoped this will be useful in the diagnosis and treatment of patients with a variety of inflammatory vascular diseases.

References

1. Bishop DK, Jutila MA, Sedmak DD, Beattie MS, Orosz CG (1989) Lymphocyte entry into inflammatory tissues in vivo. Qualitative differences of high endothelial venule-like vessels in sponge matrix allografts vs isografts. J Immunol 142:4219–4224
2. Cochrane CG, Koffler D (1973) Immune complex disease in experimental animals and man. Adv Immunol 16:185–264
3. Dustin ML, Springer T (1988) Lymphocyte function-associated antigen-1 (LFA-1) interaction with intercellular adhesion molecule-1 (ICAM-1) is one of at least three mechanisms for lymphocyte adhesion to cultured endothelial cells. J Cell Biol 107:321–331
4. Grau GE, Piguet P, Vassalli P, Lambert P (1989) Involvement of tumour necrosis factor and other cytokines in immune-mediated vascular pathology. Int Arch Allergy Appl Immunol 88:34–39
5. Guinan EC, Smith BR, Doukas JT, MIller RA, Pober JS (1989) Vascular endothelial cells enhance T cell responses by markedly augmenting IL-2 concentrations. Cell Immunol 118:166–177
6. Hart MN, Tassell SK, Sadewasser KL, Schelper RL, Moore SA (1985) Autoimmune vasculitis resulting from in vitro immunization of lymphocytes to smooth muscle. Am J Pathol 119:448–455
7. Henson PM, Johnston Jr RB (1987) Tissue injury in inflammation. Oxidants, protein-ases, and cationic proteins. J Clin Invest 79:669–674
8. Henson PM (1971) Interaction of cells with immune complexes: adherence, release of constituents, and tissue injury. J Exp Med 134:114S–135S
9. Hickey WF, Kimura H (1988) Perivascular microglial cells of the CNS are bone marrow-derived and present antigen in vivo. Science 23:290–292
10. Hughes JT, Brownell B (1966) Granulomatous giant-celled angiitis of the central nervous system. Neurology 16:293–298
11. Jirik FR, Podor TJ, Hirano T et al. (1989) Bacterial lipopolysaccharide and inflam-matory mediators augment IL-6 secretion by human endothelial cells. J Immunol 142:144–147
12. Kimani G, Tonnesen MG, Henson PM (1988) Stimulation of eosinophil adherence to human vascular endothelial cells in vitro by platelet-activated factor. J Neuroimmunol 140:3161–3166
13. Leung DYM, Geha RS, Newburger JW et al. (1986) Two monokines, interleukin 1 and tumor necrosis factor, render cultured vascular endothelial cells susceptible to lysis by antibodies circulating during kawasaki syndrome. J Exp Med 164:1958–1972
14. McIntosh RW, Koss MM (1974) The choroid plexus: immunologic injury and disease. Ann Int Med 81:111–113
15. Moore PM, Cupps TR (1983) Neurological complications of vasculitis. Ann Neurol 14:155–167

16. Moore PM (1989) Immune mechanisms in the primary and secondary vasculitides. J Neurol Sci 93:129–145
17. Moyer CF, Strandberg JD, Reinisch CL (1987) Systemic mononuclear-cell vasculitis in MRL/Mp-lpr/lpr mice. A histologic and immunocytochemical analysis. Am J Pathol 127:229-242
18. Porter DD, Larsen AE, Porter HG (1973) The Pathogenesis of Aleutian mink disease III: Immune Complex Arteritis. Am J Pathol 71:331–344
19. Stevens SK, Weissman IL, Butcher EC (1982) Differences in the migration of B and T lymphocytes: organ-selective localization in vivo and the role of lymphocyte-endothelial cell recognition. J Immunol 128:844–851
20. Van Der Woude FJ, Rasmussen N, Lobatto S et al. (1985) Autoantibodies against neutrophils and monocytes: tool for diagnosis and marker of disease activity in Wegener's granulomatosis. Lancet ii:425–429

Immunologic Diagnosis of Vasculitis

Hans H. Peter

Introduction

A variety of immunopathologic mechanisms are involved in the etiopatho-
genesis of vasculitis [1, 8]. Besides infectious agents and their immunologic
footprints, notably autoimmune diseases, malignancies, and toxic-allergic
reactions have to be considered as possible underlying causes. Numerous
attempts have been undertaken to classify vasculitides, but so far none has
been satisfactory [6]. A still widely accepted scheme distinguishes *primary
and secondary vasculitides,* although new classifications according to immunologic parameters (e.g., antinuclear antibody, ANA-, or antineutrophilic
cytoplasmic autoantibody, ANCA-positive, hyper-, hypo-, or normocomple-
mentemic vasculitis) may soon prevail. Table 1 summarizes the most frequent vasculitis syndromes and some of the associated key laboratory findings. In Table 2 an attempt is made to group vasculitides into ANCA
positive, ANA positive and ANCA/ANA negative ones.

2 The Clinical Approach

Any clinical suspicion of vasculitis requires a thorough medical history to be
taken, including family and personal history, habits, and occupation (Table
3). Subsequently a careful *physical examination* followed by a *diagnostic
screening program* as shown in Table 4 are mandatory. The listed tests
should not be performed rigidly but rather adapted to the individual needs
of each patient. Diagnostic hallmarks in vasculitis are a variety of bacterial,
viral, autoantigen, and drug-related antibodies. Furthermore, circulating
immune complexes, complement split products (C3a, C3d), and acute phase
proteins (C-reactive protein, fibrinogen, ferritin, haptoglobin, C3), as well
as paraproteins, cryoglobulin, and cryofibrinogen have to be considered.

3 The Immunologic Approach

The clinical manifestations of vasculitis depend on the type of antigen
involved (autoantigen, foreign antigen), the predominant immunopatho-

P. Berlit, P. M. Moore (Eds.)
Vasculitis, Rheumatic Disease
and the Nervous System
© Springer-Verlag Berlin Heidelberg 1993

Table 1. Conventional classification of vasculitis syndromes

Type of vasculitis	Diagnostic Features
I. Primary Vasculitides	
1. Small vessel vasculitis (SVV) (hypersensitivity angiitis)	IC, cryoglobulins, CH_{50}, C3d, ANA, ANCA, antimicrobial and antidrug Abs
2. Periarteritis nodosa	
a) Classical form (cPAN)	IC, APP, HBsAg, AST, ANCA, endothelial toxins, etc
b) Microscopic form (mPAN)	pANCA/anti-MPO Ab, APP
c) Kawasaki's disease (KS)	APP, antiendothelial Ab, ANCA
3. Granulomatous vasculitis	
a) Wegener's granulomatosis (WG)	cANCA/anti-PR3 Ab, APP
b) Churg–Strauss syndrome	Eosinophilia, IgE, cANCA, APP, IC
c) Isolated angiitis of CNS (IAC)	?, leptomeningeal biopsy
d) Behçet's disease (BD)	
4. Giant cell arteritis	
a) Takayasu's arteritis	APP, CRP-induced complement activation
b) Temporal arteritis (TA)	APP, antielastin Ab
c) Polymyalgia rheumatica (PMR)	APP, CRP-induced complement activation
II. Secondary vasculitides	
1. Collagen vascular and rheumatic diseases	
a) Systemic lupus erythematosus, mixed connective tissue disease, progressive systemic sclerosis	ANA, CH_{50}, C3, C4, C3d, IC
b) Phospholipid antibody syndrome	Anticardiolipin Ab, C3d
c) Rheumatoid arthritis (RA)	RF, cryoglobulins, APP
d) Still's disease	?, APP, IC
e) Thrombangiitis obliterans	?, CRP, antielastin Ab
2. Para- and postinfectious vasculitis	
a) Hepatitis B	HBsAg, Anti-HBc, Anti-HBe
b) Rheumatic fever	Streptococcal Ab
c) Borreliosis	Anti-*Borrelia* Ab
d) Syphilis	VDRL Ab
e) Parasitoses (kala-azar, etc.)	Leishmanial Ab
f) Viral infections	EBV, CMV, HIV, etc.
3. Malignant diseases	
a) Monoclonal gammopathy	Paraproteins, cryoglobulins
b) Angioimmunoblastic LAP	Multiple autoantibodies
c) Leukemia, lymphoma	Coagulopathy, APP, cytokines
d) Small lung cell carcinoma	APP, C3d, IgA, cytokines
e) Atrial myxoma	Cytokines (IL-6), embolism
4. Drug-related allergic vasculitis	
a) Erythema multiforme	APP, specific antidrug Ab
b) Drug-induced lupus erythematosus	Antihistone Ab

Abbreviations: ?, no typical serologic test available; Ab, antibody; ANA, antinuclear antibody; ANCA, antineutrophilic cytoplasmic antibody; APP, acute phase proteins; cANCA, classic ANCA; CMV, cytomegalovirus; CRP, C-reactive protein; EBV, Epstein-Barr virus; HBc, hepatitis B core; HBsAg, hepatitis B surface antigen; HBe, hepatitis B "e" antigen; HIV, human immunodeficiency virus; IC, immune complexes; IL, interleukin; MPO, myeloperoxidase; PR3 proteinase 3; pANCA, perinuclear ANCA; RF, rheumatoid factor.

Table 2. Immunologic classification of vasculitides

ANCA positive vasculitides
Wegener's syndrome (WG)
Churg-Strauss syndrome (CSS)
Microscopic polyarteritis (mPAN)
Crescent forming rapid progressive GN (RPGN)
Kawasaki syndrome (KS)
Classic polyarteritis nodosa (cPAN)

ANA positive vasculitides
Systemic lupus erythematosus (SLE)
Mixed connective tissue disease (MCTD)
Progressive systemic sclerosis (PSS)
Extraarticular rheumatoid arthritis (RA)
Secondary Sjögren's syndrome (SS)
Overlap syndromes

ANCA/ANA negative vasculitides
Classic polyarteritis nodosa
Behcet's disease (BD)
Schönlein Hennoch purpura
Giant cell arteriitis: Takayasu Syndrome
                      Temporal arteritis (TA)
Isolated angiitis of the CNS
Thromboangiitis obliterans
Allergic vasculitis
Post- and parainfectious vasculitis
Paraneoplastic vasculitis
Cryoglobulinemia / Cryofibrinogenemia

Table 3. Vasculitis-related medical history

Family history	Rheumatic disease, hyperlipidemia, diabetes
Personal history	Recent infections, tick bites
	Effects of cold and warmth
	Weight loss, fatigue, sweating, Raynaud's phenomenon, livedo reticularis or racemosa
	Diabetes, hyperlipidemia, hyperuricemia
	Rheumatic and collagen vascular disease
	Allergies
	Renal disease, hypertension
	Malignancies
	Trauma
Habits	Smoking, alcohol, drug abuse
	Contraceptive pills
	Any medication
	Pets
Occupation	Increased exposured to cold, pressure, vibration, chemicals, heavy metals

Table 4. Vasculitis diagnostic screening program

Routine laboratory tests	– Erythrocyte sedimentation rate, blood formula, lipids, – Liver and kidney funtion tests, lactate dehydrogenase, electrophoresis, CK – Proteinuria, glucosuria, disk electrophoresis – Clotting tests; Quick, partial thromboplastin time (PTT), thrombine time (TZ), factor VIII, platelet aggregation, fibrinogen split products
Culture	Blood, urine, stool, throat, spinal fluid
Viral antibodies	HBV, CMV, EBV, HIV, HSV, HCV, etc.
Bacterial antibodies	Streptococci, *Yersinia, Salmonella, Chlamydia, Borrelia, Mycoplasma,* etc.
Fungal antibodies	*Aspergillus, Candida,* etc.
Protein pathology	Quantitative IgG, A, E, M, paraproteins, cryoglobulins, cryofibrinogen
Autoantibodies	ANA, ANCA, antiphospholipid antibodies, RF, AMA, SMA, lupus anticoagulans, cold agglutinins
Complement	CH_{50}, C3, C_4, C3d, immune complexes, C1qlNH, CRP-mediated complement activation
Acute phase proteins	CRP, fibrinogen, haptoglobin, ferritin
Imaging	Chest X-ray, abdominal and cardiac echography, cranial CT, MRI, angiography, etc.

Abbreviations: Ab, antibody; AMA, antimitochondrial antibody; ANA, antinuclear antibody; ANCA, antineutrophilic cytoplasmic antibody; C1qINH, C1q esterase inhibitor; CMV, cytomegalovirus; CRP, C-reactive protein; CT, computed tomography; EBV, Epstein–Barr virus; HCV, hepatitis C virus; HBV, hepatitis B virus; HIV, human immunodeficiency virus; HSV, herpes simplex virus; MRI, magnetic resonance imaging; RF, rheumatoid factor; SMA, smooth muscle antibodies.

Table 5. Type I reactions

Laboratory findings	Vasculitic syndromes
Eosinophilia	Churg–Strauss syndrome (CSS) Eosinophilia–myalgia syndrome
Total IgE elevated	Polyarteritis nodosa (classic, cPAN, and microscropic, mPAN) Wegener's granulomatosis (WG)
IgE-containing immune complexes	Churg–Strauss syndrome, parasitosis
Specific IgE elevated	Allergic reactions, parasitosis, drugs

logic reaction induced (types I–IV), and associated conditions (e.g., age, sex, other diseases, pregnancy, drugs). In Tables 5–10 an attempt has been made to associate immunopathologic reactions types I–IV of Coombs and Gell to immunologic findings (antigens, antibodies, laboratory tests) in the various forms of vasculitis listed in Table 1. The immunologic approach to vasculitis does not claim to be superior to any other classification scheme; it simply tries to associate clinical knowledge on certain vasculitides with an established immunopathologic framework [7].

Table 6. Type II reactions

Targets	Laboratory tests	Vasculitis
Erythrocytes	Cold agglutinins	Cold agglutinin disease: idiopathic or postinfectious (*Mycoplasma,* Epstein–Barr virus)
Granulocytes	cANCA (PR3)	Wegener's granulomatosis, classic and microscopic polyarteritis nodosa
	pANCA (MPO)	Microscopic polyarteritis nodosa, RPGN
	xANCA (?)	Colitis ulcerosa
Thrombocytes	Antiphospholipid Ab	Sneddon's syndrome, systemic lupus erythematosus
Endothelial cells	Cytokine induced antigens	Kawasaki's syndrome

Ab, antibody; cANCA, classic antineutrophilic cytoplasmic antibody; pANCA, perinuclear ANCA; xANCA, undefined ANCA; MPO, myeloperoxidase; PR3, proteinase 3; RPGN, rapidly progressive glomerulonephritis.

Table 7. Type III reactions: Immune complexes involving autoantigens

Autoantigens	Vasculitic syndromes
ANA, dsDNA, U1-sRNP, Topo I	SLE, MCTD, PSS
Centromere, Ro, LA	CREST, Sjögren's syndrome
Cytoplasmic mitochondria	PBC
Cytochrome pb 450s	Autoimmune hepatitis
Proteinase 3	Wegener's granulomatosis
Myeloperoxidase	mPAN, RPGN
Cathepsin G?	Colitis ulcerosa, primary sclerosing cholangitis
Immunoglobulins (rheumatoid factor)	Rheumatoid arthritis
Cryoglobulins	Small vessel vasculitis, mPAN, cPAN, SLE, rheumatoid arthritis, PBC, etc.
Cryofibrinogens	Paraneoplastic disease, thrombosis
Phospholipids	Sneddon's syndrome, SLE
Collagen II	Rheumatoid arthritis, polychondritis
Heat shock proteins	Reactive arthritis?
Hormones	Thyroiditis, type I diabetes

ANA, antinuclear antibody; cPAN, mPAN, classic and microscopic polyarteritis nodosa; LA, nuclear antigen SS-B; MCTD, mixed connective tissue disease; PBC, primary biliary cirrhosis; PSS, progressive systemic sclerosis; Ro, nuclear antigen SS-A; RPGN, rapidly progressive glomerulonephritis; SLE, systemic lupus erythematosus; U1-snRNP, small nuclear ribonucleoprotein; Topo I, topoisomerase I.

Type I reactions represent immunoglobulin E- (IgE-)mediated immune phenomena. Among the vasculititides which show elevated serum IgE levels and/or eosinophilia, the allergic granulomatosis Churg-Strauss, the ANCA-positive vasculitides, and drug- and parasite-induced reactions must be considered. As modern cellular immunology distinguishes T_{H1} and T_{H2} immune reactions, it should be stressed that T_{H2} cells preferentially produce inter-

Table 8. Type III reactions: Immune complexes involving foreign antigens

Foreign antigens	Vasculitic syndromes
Bacterial antigens	
Yersinia enterocolitica 03	*Reactive arthritis*
Chlamydia trachomatis	Reactive arthritis
Streptococcal antigen	Rheumatic fever, Still's disease
Borrelia burgdorferi	Lyme disease
Treponema pallidum	Syphilis
Viral antigens	
Small vessel vasculitis	
Epstein–Barr virus	Mononucleosis
Cytomegalovirus	Mononucleosis-like disease
Herpes simplex virus	Skin, CNS lesions
Parasitic antigens	Kala azar
Fungal antigens	Mycotic vasculitis

Table 9. Type III reactions: Immune complexes involving drugs

Drugs	Vasculitic syndromes
Penicillin	Generalized vasculitis, variably associated
Sulfonamides	with:
Pyrazolone	– Erythema multiforme
Nonsteroidal antiinflammatory drugs	– Alveolitis, pneumonitis
Allopurinol	– Hepatitis
Carbamazepine	– Nephritis
Amiodarone	– Myositis, arthritis
Hydantoin	– Agranulocytosis
Methotrexate	– Fever, eosinophilia
Furantoin	
Procainamide, hydralazin, isoniazid, hydantoin, D-penicillamine, quinidine, methyldopa	Drug-induced systemic lupus erythematosus
Foreign proteins (e.g., monoclonal antibodies)	Serum sickness
Dextran gamma-Globulins Food additives	Anaphylaxia with urticaria or angioedema and shock
Insulin	Local necrosis (Arthus)

Table 10. Type IV reactions

Antigens	Vasculitic syndromes
Lysosomal enzymes	
Proteinase 3	Wegener's granulomatosis
Myeloperoxidase, elastase?	Polyarteritis nodosa (microscopic, classic), rapidly progressive glomerulonephritis
Cathepsin G?	Colitis ulcerosa
Elastic fibers?	Giant cell arteritis
Drugs	
Antibiotics	Eczema, erythroderma
Gold	Eczema, nephritis
Bacterial, viral, fungal, and parasitic antigens	Granulomatous and necrotizing vasculitis

leukin 4 (IL-4), a T-cell switch factor for IgE production, and IL-5, which induces eosinophilia (Table 5) [3, 4].

Type II reactions are characterized by the presence of antibodies binding to cell surfaces and inducing either complement- and/or effector cell-mediated lysis. In the vascular endothelium, cells that are innocent bystanders (endothelium and smooth muscle cells) may be damaged by activated complement components, immune complexes, platelet-activating factor (PAF), and lysosomal enzymes. Type II reactions leading to vasculitis lesions may be encountered in ANCA-positive vasculitides, cold agglutinin disease, and conditions associated with antiphospholipid and antiendothelial cell autoantibodies [2, 5] (Table 6).

Type III reactions represent immune complex-mediated tissue damage and vascular lesions. Increased production or impaired clearance of circulating immune complexes leads to activation of granulocytes, macrophages, and thrombocytes; endothelial damage and immune complex deposition in tissues may ensue [7]. Typical examples are immune complex nephritis in systemic lupus erythematosus, leukocytoclastic vasculitis, allergic bronchiolitis and serum sickness. Type III reactions have long been considered to be the only relevant immunopathologic reaction in vasculitis. Tables 7–9 summarize immune complex reactions involving the most frequent foreign antigens, autoantigens, and drugs. Whereas the antigenic trigger may be highly variable in immune complex-induced vasculitis, the histopathologic outcome is rather uniform; one sees either small vessel vasculitis of capillaries and postcapillary venules or necrotizing vasculitis involving small arteries. Depending on the organs involved more or less severe disease manifestations may result.

Type IV reactions are characterized by cellular infiltrates typical for delayed-type hypersensitivity. The histopathologic correlates are tuberculoid and sarcoid lesions, rheumatoid nodules, and granulomatous and giant cell arteritis. Activated macrophages, histiocytes, giant cells, and lymphocytes dominate the cellular infiltrate. Current concepts of T-cell immunology consider type IV reactions as T_{H1}-mediated conditions which involve the cytokines IL-2 and γ-interferon [3, 4]. In vasculitis lesions T cells may react with autoantigens such as lysosomal enzymes (proteinase 3, myeloperoxidase, elastase, etc.), elastic fibers (giant cell arteritis), collagen, and alloantigens. In secondary vasculitides, drugs (e.g., gold, d-penicillamine, antibiotics, pyrazolones) and microbial antigens may be the target structures for a delayed-type hypersensitivity reaction (Table 10).

Most clinically evident vasculitides are mixtures of different immunopathologic reactions with one prevailing type. Thus, Wegener's granulomatosis is characterized by type IV-like granulomatous tissue infiltrates and classic antineutrophilic cytoplasmic autoantibody (cANCA) capable of inducing a type II reaction. In allergic granulomatosis Churg–Strauss high concentrations of serum IgE- and IgE-containing immune complexes indicate type I and III reactions, whereas the granulomatous infiltrates of the lung show features of a type IV reaction. The factors and conditions which are ultimately responsible for the immunopathologic outcome in vasculitis are manyfold and far from being clear. The type of antigen, the immunogenetic background of the host, the cytokine network, accompanying diseases, and environmental factors are all likely to play a role.

References

1. Hunder GG, et al. (1991) Vasculitic syndromes. Curr Opin Rheumatol 3:1–56
2. Lockshin MD (1991) Antiphospholipid antibody and antiphospholipid antibody syndrome. Curr Opin Rheumatol 3:797–802
3. Mossmann TR, Coffman RL (1989) Heterogeneity of cytokine secretion patterns and functions of helper T cells. Adv Immunol 45:107
4. Mossmann TR, Moore KW (1991) The role of IL-10 in crossregulation of TH1 and TH2 responses. Immunoparasitol Today 12:49–53
5. Mountz JD, Gause WC, Jonsson R (1991) Murine models for systemic lupus erythematosus and Sjögren's syndrome. Curr Opin Rheumatol 3:738–756
6. Peter HH (1991) Vaskulitiden. In: Peter HH (ed) Klinische Immunologie. Innere Medizin der Gegenwart, vol 9. Urban and Schwarzenberg, Munich, pp 411–414
7. Stadler BM, de Weck AL (1991) Allergie. In: Gemsa D, Kalden JR, Resch K (eds) Immunologie – Grundlagen, Klinik und Praxis, 3rd edn. Thieme, Stuttgart, pp 216–231
8. Wolff K, Winkelmann RK (1980) Vasculitis. Lloyd-Luke, London

Magnetic Resonance Imaging and Angiography in Vasculitides of the Central Nervous System

Andreas Schwartz

1 Introduction

Magnetic resonance imaging (MRI) and angiography are synergistic diagnostic methods that together can often provide clues to lesions that are beyond the abilities of each procedure alone. MRI is a tomographic method which produces a layered picture of the brain parenchyma in three image dimensions: the parenchyma of the brain is illustrated. Angiography involves projection through a contrast medium. The contours of the contrast medium-filled vessels are projected via the exposure of the plain X-ray film or the digital image intensifier: changes in the arteries and veins are visualized indirectly. Magnetic resonance angiography (MRA), which uses the flowing protons of the blood to produce a three-dimensional display of the vessel, has been discussed as an alternative to conventional angiography but its resolution is much lower than that of conventional angiography or even of the currently common digital substraction angiography (DSA): the conventional plain-film technique can discriminate 5 line pairs/mm, while DSA with a 512×512 matrix can resolve 2 line pairs/mm, and MRA is only capable of resolving approximately 0.5 line pairs/mm, assuming that a sequence is chosen which works with a normal duration of measurement and a 254×256 matrix.

Figures 1–3 show how the details that can be perceived decrease as the reolution decreases in the ratio 5:2:0.5. While plain-film angiography (Fig. 1) shows pathologic vessel wall alterations of the intracranial vessels behind the A2, M2, and P2 segments, arterial DSA (Fig. 2) cannot resolve the changes in these segments. Although MRA (Fig. 3) has surprisingly good resolution of the large vessels of the circle of Willis, the smaller arteries of the periphery cannot be followed, in contrast to the clear visualization by DSA (Fig. 2). This is most clearly seen in the opacification of the ophthalmic artery (Figs. 2, 3). An improvement in the resolution can be attained in modern instruments by increasing the matrix from 128×128 to 256×256 or even 512×512 (Fig. 4). However, the resolving power of DSA can not be as good as that of plain film series. In MRA increasing the matrix almost doubles the examination time, thus aggravating problems due to movement artifacts.

P. Berlit, P. M. Moore (Eds.)
Vasculitis, Rheumatic Disease
and the Nervous System
© Springer-Verlag Berlin Heidelberg 1993

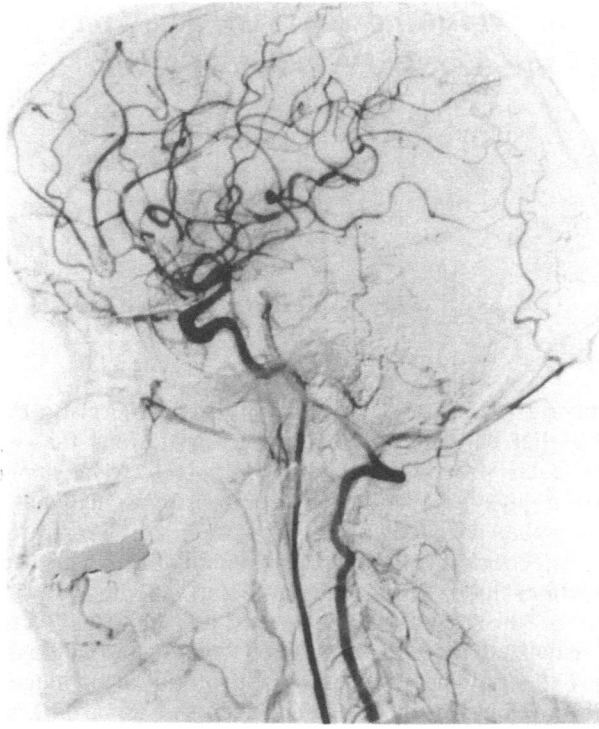

Fig. 1. Plain-film angiography: resolution about 5 line pairs/mm

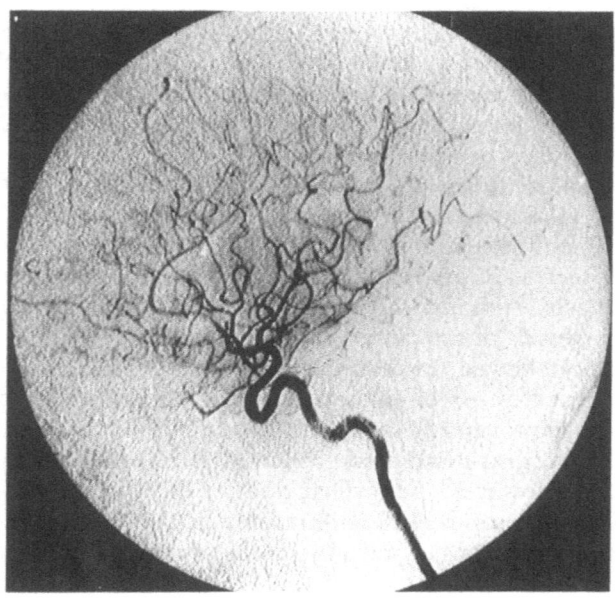

Fig. 2. Arterial DSA: resolution about 2 line pairs/mm

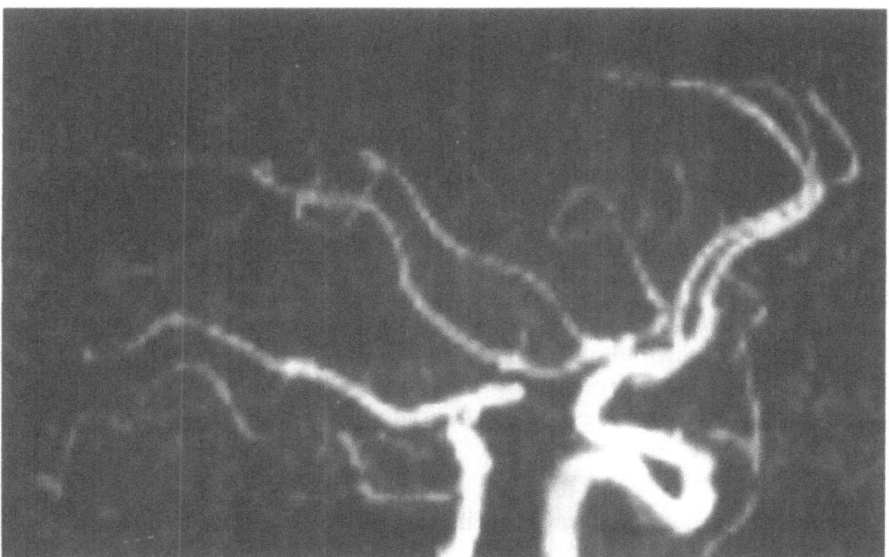

Fig. 3. MRA: resolution about 0.5 line pairs/mm

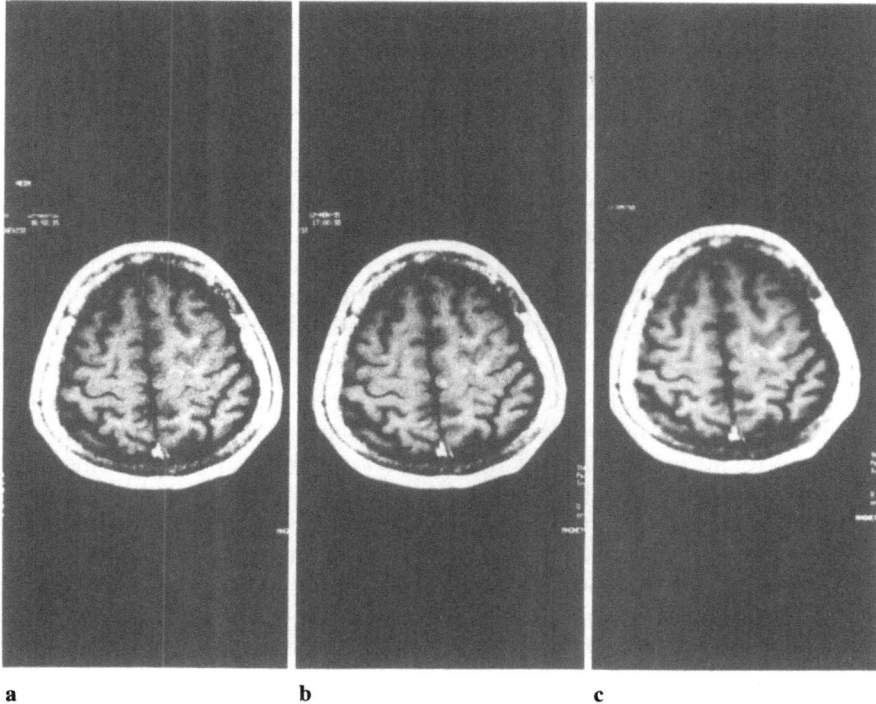

a   b   c

Fig. 4 a–c. MRA with matrices of **a** 128 × 128, **b** 256 × 256, and **c** 512 × 512

2 Angiography in Vasculitis

A review of the literature on angiography [8, 13, 14, 16] shows clearly that arteritis is most often described but reports on inflammatory changes of the venous system are sparse, and changes of the arterioles or the capillaries cannot be resolved satisfactorily by angiography. MRI may give us more information on the perivascular tissue. Only a relatively small number of vasculitides present with a purely or predominantly cerebral manifestation. This chapter focusses on temporal arteritis, Churg–Strauss syndrome, lymphomatoid granulomatosis, Wegener's granulomatosis, polyarteritis nodosa, and the neuroradiologic appearance of systemic lupus erythematosus.

From the neuroradiologic point of view, only two angiographic criteria exist by which the different disorders may be distinguished:
1. the site of vascular lesion and the type of vessel involved, and
2. the angiographic appearance of the vessel alterations.

Furthermore, the angiographer will only be able to identify a small fraction of the vessel wall changes known to occur from pathology studies. Thus, relatively few consistent vessel wall alterations are angiographically documented. The following changes may be seen angiographically in vasculitis [5, 8, 11, 16]:
1. Vasoparalysis with dilated vessel segments, which produces stasis of the contrast medium during the angiogram series.
2. Vasospasms, sometimes localized, sometimes over longer segments with concentric narrowing of the vessel. The vessel wall stays smooth and sometimes the stenosis has an hourglass appearance.
3. Necrotizing vessel alterations with circumscribed vessel wall pouches, which may lead to pseudoaneurysms. The inflammatory process can lead to an intimal swelling of the vessel wall with narrowing of the lumen. Consequently, stenosed and dilated segments can be found side by side.
4. Proliferative arteritis, which results in thickening of the vessel wall with nodules, leading to irregularly shaped, moniliform stenoses.

This mixed, atypically located pattern may allow vasculitis to be distinguished from intracranial atherosclerosis, because the atherosclerotic changes are found predominantly at the vessel divisions. A very specific pattern is found in intracranial infectious arteritis, where changes develop only in specific segments. The vasoparalytic dilatations or the inflammatory stenoses are found frequently along those vessel segments lying in the subarachnoid space where the infection has a special space to spread into [9].

Both the topology and the morphology of the vessel wall alterations seen on angiography may allow classification of the disorder into one of the subgroups of vasculitis before a biopsy is used to verify the diagnosis. The following angiographic description of vasculitic vessel wall changes follows the topologic approach from extracranial to intracranial.

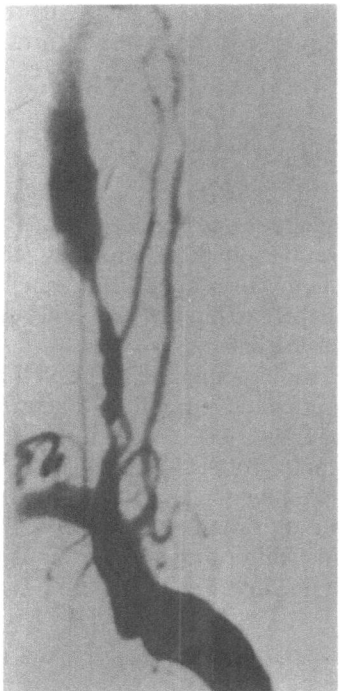
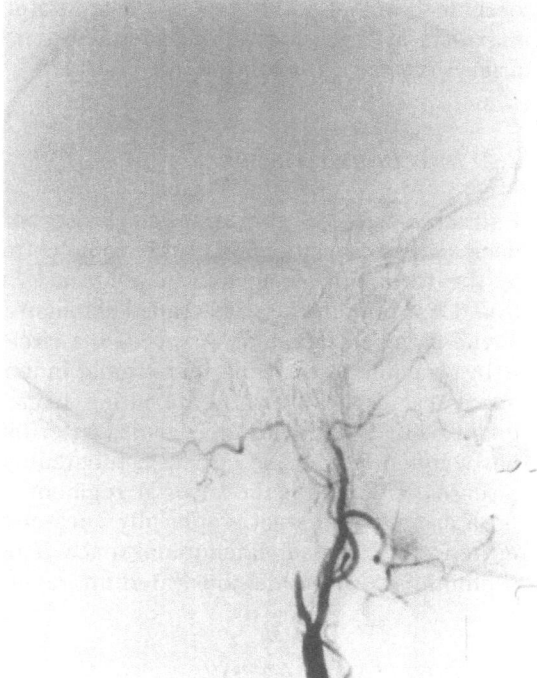

Fig. 5. Takayasu's arteritis: concentric stenoses of the lumen and obstruction of the aorta of the smaller vessels

Fig. 6. Temporal arteritis: multiple occlusions

2.1 Giant Cell Arteritis

Giant cell arteritis comprises two diseases of the large arteries: Takayasu's arteritis and temporal arteritis. Takayasu's arteritis starts at the aortic arch and spreads along the aorta as well as into the supraaortic branches, following the extracranial vessels up to the skull base [12, 13]. Temporal arteritis is localized predominantly in the external carotid system, with some involvement of intracranial vessels, particularly the posterior circulation [7].

In Takayasu's arteritis, inflammation leads to a concentric stenosis of the lumen over a longer distance with obstruction of the ostia of the smaller vessels (Fig. 5). Theoretically, MRI with transverse slices in T2-weighted spin-echo sequences should be able to demonstrate thickening of the vessel walls with high signal intensity.

Temporal or cranial arteritis may lead to occlusions of the vessels involved via secondary thrombosis in segments with inflammatory changes of the intima or reactive intima fibrosis. In the example in Fig. 6, multiple occlusions can be seen. Not only is the opening of the internal carotid artery occluded, but also the superficial temporal artery; this contrasts with the maxillary artery, which, alongside the other branches of the external carotid artery, is filled with contrast medium.

2.2 Infectious Arteritis

Extracranial vessel alterations may also be seen in *infectious arteritis*. The necrotic vessel wall changes in chronic extracranial inflammations may lead to the formation of mycotic aneurysms. Such mycotic aneurysms can be found not only in the extracranial segments of the carotid arteries, but also in the larger intracranial vessels of the circle of Willis.

In principle, any of the intracranial inflammations – meningitis as well as abscesses, especially those resulting from septicemic emboli in bacterial endocarditis – can lead to arteritis. Arteritis of the basal intracranial vessels has frequently been described in tuberculosis and syphilis [4, 5, 9]. In both diseases, frequently the arterial segments that haved passed through the dura are affected angiographically. Vessel wall alterations begin just at the entrance into the subarachnoidal space. This distribution of stenotic signs in syphilitic arteritis is demonstrated impressively in Figure 7.

2.3 Intracranial Arteritis

Intracranial arteritis may be a presentation of polyarteritis nodosa, Churg-Strauss allergic granulomatosis, Wegener's granulomatosis, hypersensitivity arteritis, isolated angiitis of the CNS, and vasculitis in collagen vascular diseases. In most diseases, medium- and small-sized vessels are primarily involved. Only the changes of the arteries can be detected by angiography, even when plain-film techniques are employed.

Polyarteritis nodosa (Fig. 8) presents with a segmental pattern of vessel narrowings and occlusions in the periphery (Fig. 8a). High magnification (Fig. 8b) can elucidate these changes. Angiography reveals segments with stenoses together with parts which are dilated. In other cases (e.g., Fig. 9) the segmental pattern of the stenoses and the occlusions are not as clearly visible. Differentiation of the vasculitides on the basis of the angiographic appearance of the vessel wall changes is not possible [1, 2].

In *secondary vasculitides,* occlusions in the large vessels at the base of the scull may be found in a very early stage of the disease (Fig. 10). The collateral blood supply of the cortical arteries is established via small "moya-moya"-like capillary networks originating from the deep perforating arteries or leptomeningeal anastomoses from the meningeal arteries. This collateral pattern, together with the bilateral stenoses or occlusions of the carotid arteries, may be caused by infections such as herpes-zoster meningoence-phalitis in the young. The "moya-moya syndrome" may result from a large variety of occlusive angiopathies at the scull base (e.g., radiation lesions,

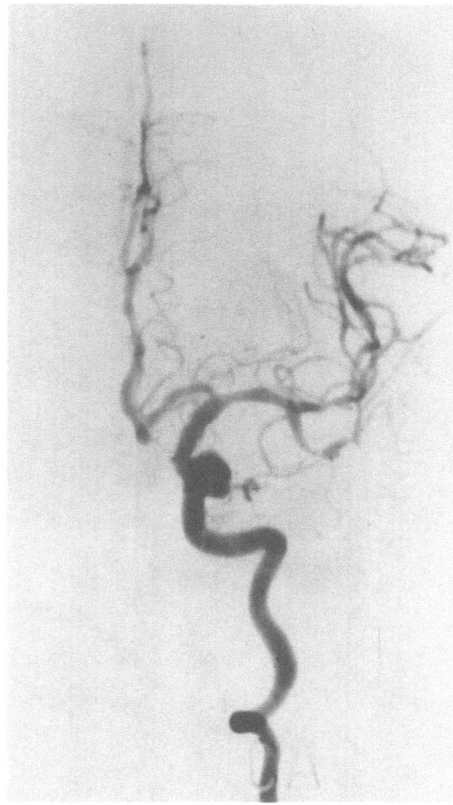

Fig. 7. Syphilitic arteritis: the stenotic signs

atherosclerosis). Hypertrophy of the deep perforating vessels and other short circuits originating from the anterior or medial cerebral artery for collateral blood supply has nothing to do with the typical neogenesis of vessels in moya-moya disease (Fig. 11). A definite relationship between this disorder and vasculitic disorders has still not been found [6].

3 Magnetic Resonance Imaging

Magnetic resonance imaging (MRI) techniques enable us to obtain special projections of the vessels by means of gradient-echo sequences comparable to those of conventional angiography. Early results show that magnetic resonance angiography (MRA) is a reliable method for detecting the site of stenoses, but it still has problems in identifying the morphologic configuration of the stenosis. As the method is dependent on the flow in the vessel, only high-grade stenoses can be found with any sort of confidence, and

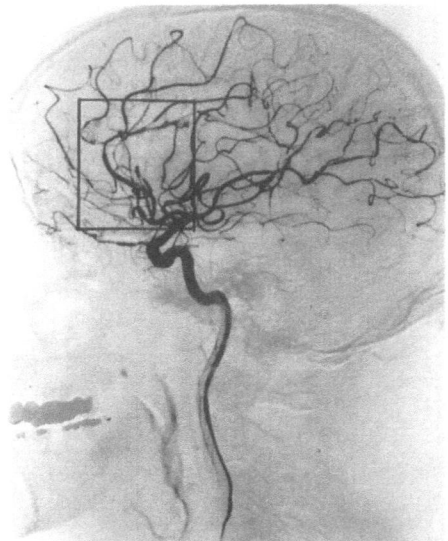

a

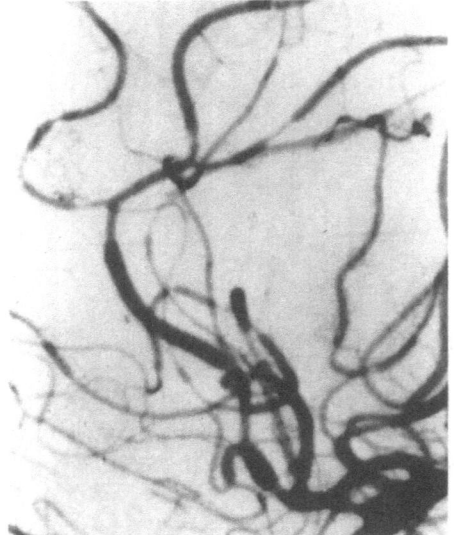

b

Fig. 8a, b. Polyarteritis nodosa.
a Segmental pattern of narrowings and
occlusions. **b** Higher magnification

subtotal stenoses or occlusions cannot be differentiated. On this basis, MRA has no place in the diagnostic repertoire for vasculitis.

On the other hand, MRI-slices using the spin-echo technique with T2-, proton-, and T1-weighted images are able to detect possible changes in the affected tissue. In *infectious vasculitis,* for instance, extended edema of the white matter or brain abscesses can be visualized, along with vessel occlu-

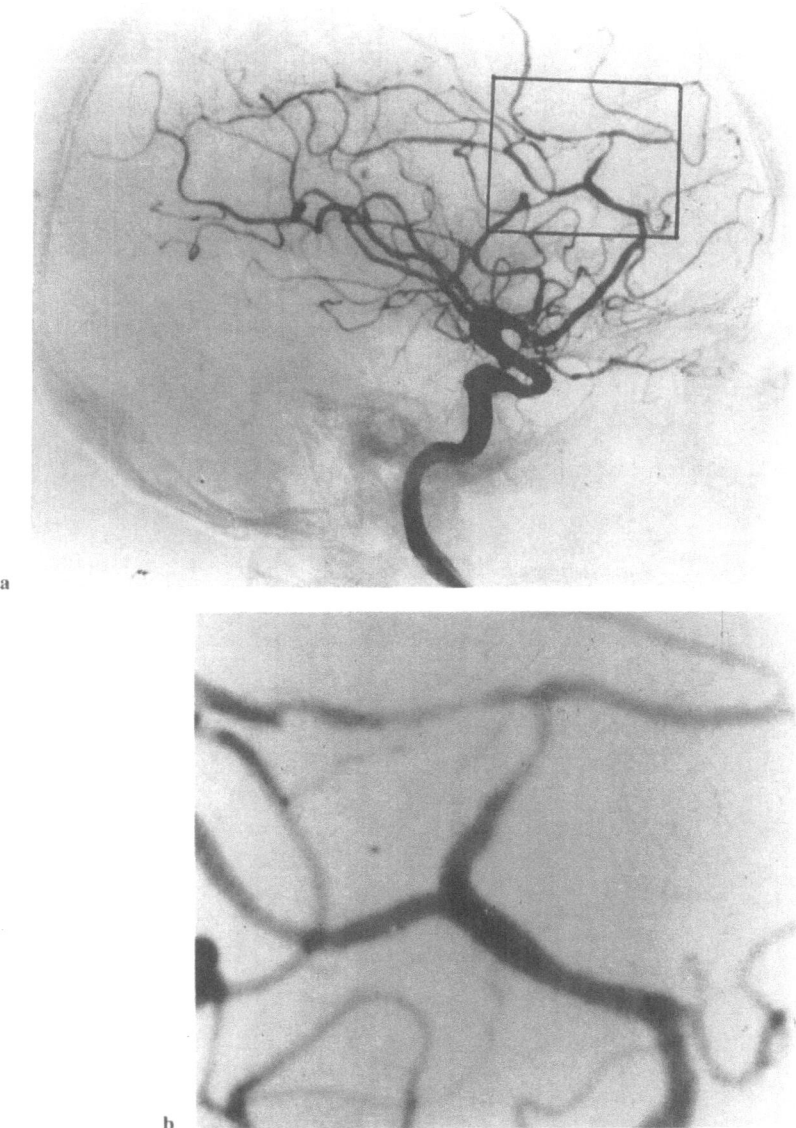

Fig. 9a, b. Polyarteritis nodosa: the segmental pattern is not as clearly visible

sions, because of the typical pattern of lesions along the vascular boundaries. In the first stage these infarcts can only be seen in T2- and proton-weighted images. Later they present with the well-demarcated borders of pseudocystic lesions. This development is accompanied by signal enhancement in T2-weighted images.

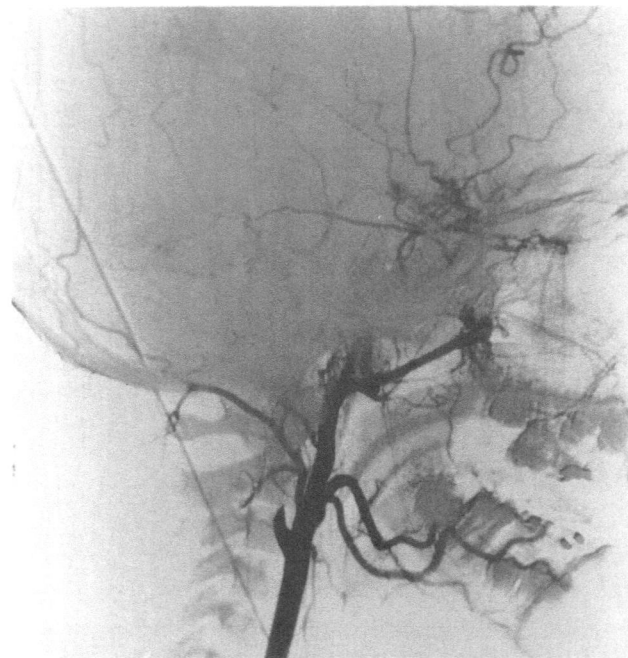

Fig. 10. Infectious vasculitis: occlusions of the large vessels at the skull base

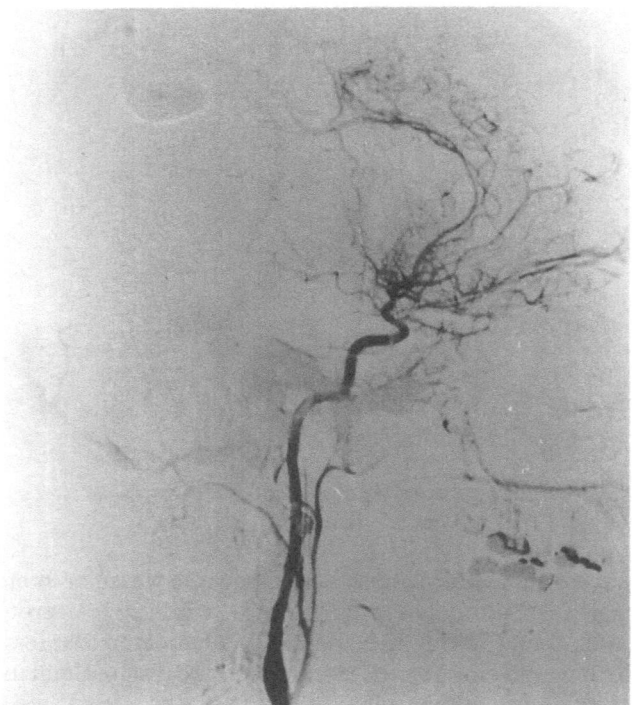

Fig. 11. Moya-moya: the typical neogenesis of vessels

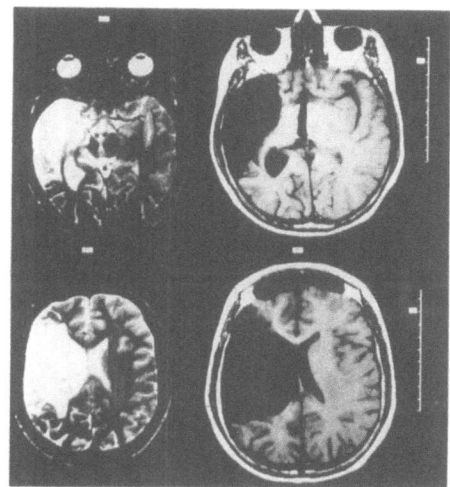

Fig. 12. Systemic lupus erythematosus:
middle cerebral artery infarction

In one of our patients with *systemic lupus erythematosus* (SLE) (Fig. 12), the middle cerebral artery infarction was not caused by an intracranial vascular process, but by an emboligenic occlusion. This embolus resulted from the associated Libmann–Sacks endocarditis [3]. Large-vessel vasculitis in SLE is a rare event [15].

Looking for the inflammatory substrate of collagen vascular disease, we found in T2- and proton-weighted images small, pin-point-shaped, signal-intense foci in the subcortical white matter of neuro-SLE patients (Fig. 13). It is typical of these cases that the foci cannot be recognized in the corresponding T1-weighted images [3]. Consequently, they cannot be pseudocystic defects. In some rare cases signal enhancement can be found after intravenous injection of paramagnetic contrast medium in the T1-weighted image. In those cases, an acute inflammation may be postulated as the background. This interpretation is supported by the observation that these foci appear and fade away during follow-up examinations, especially after specific therapy. Sometimes the contrast enhancement is diminished by the therapy.

The example of another patient with SLE (Fig. 14a) shows a slight signal loss in the right frontocentral focus in T2-weighted images after 20 months of therapy. Meanwhile, two other lesions (Fig. 14b) had appeared in the frontal lobe, one in the frontobasal and one in the frontopolar region. These are examples of lesions which can be found not only in collagen vascular disease but also in other conditions. However, it must be pointed out that those foci do not follow any of the known vascular patterns which lead to typical defects. In a high number of cases the foci heal without any signal change, while in others they show the same signal intensity in T2- and proton-density-weighted images over years.

In our experience, there is no relation between the location of the lesions and the clinical symptoms. In a retrospective study of 32 patients with SLE

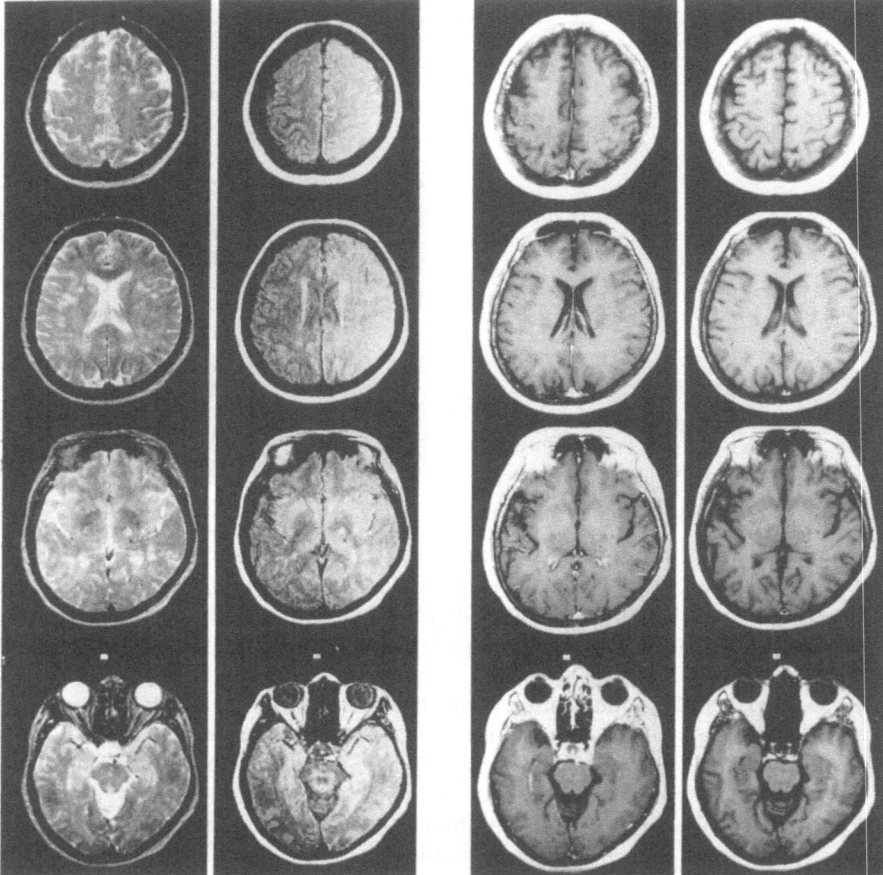

Fig. 13 a, b. Neurologic systemic lupus erythematosus: small, signal-intense foci in the subcortical white matter

and neurologic or psychiatric symptoms, no correlation was found between the MRI or computed tomography lesion and the clinically assumed site of the defect [3].

4 Conclusions

After a tentative diagnosis of vasculitis has been made, angiography has the task of demonstrating pathologic vessel wall alterations and MRI is used to delineate focal tissue changes. The identification of vessel wall changes or of a focus on MRI alone does not allow vasculitis to be diagnosed. For precise evaluation of vasculitic lesions only plain-film angiography or DSA with a 1024 × 1024 matrix are adequate techniques. Only the vessel alterations in

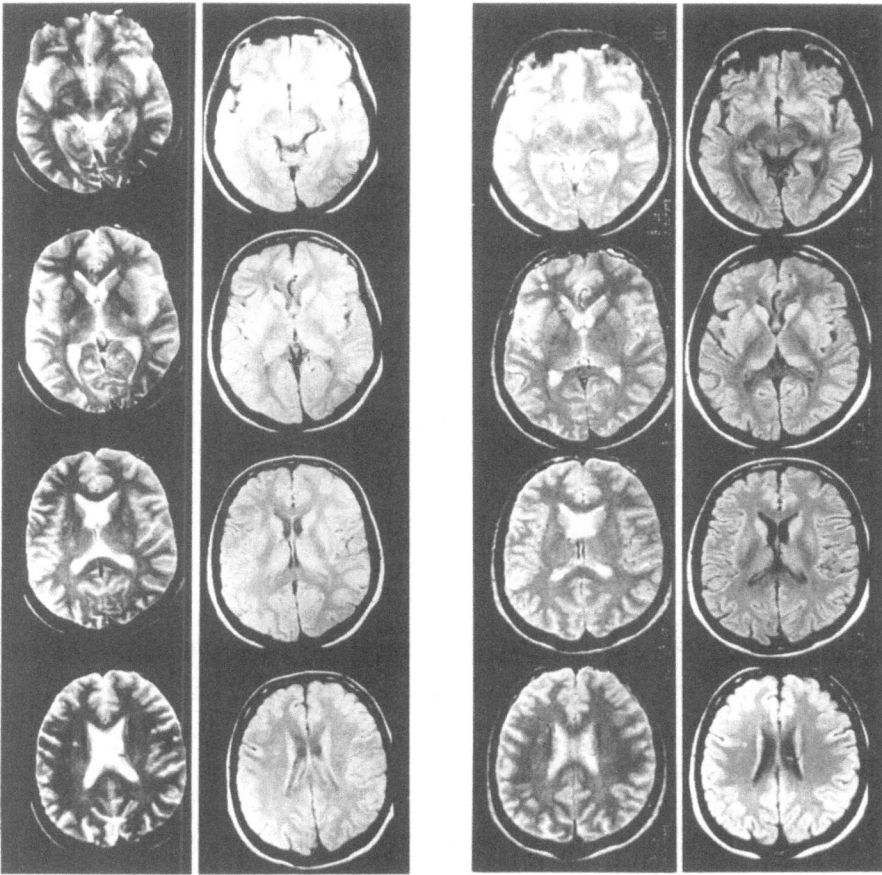

Fig. 14a, b. Systemic lupus erythematosus: signal loss in the right frontocentral focus (**a**) and appearance of new frontobasal and frontopolar lesions (**b**)

the extracranial region may be examined by alternative techniques with lower resolutions.

Knowing the topography of the vascular lesions and the type and size of the vessels involved helps in the diagnosis of vasculitis syndromes. Depending on the underlying disease, the extracranial arteries, the larger vessels of the circle of Willis, the vessels along the subarachnoid space, or the smaller arterioles in the brain parenchyma may be predominantly affected. In general, it is possible to differentiate between vasculitis and intracranial atherosclerosis. The diagnostic value of angiography – it confirms the diagnosis of vasculitis in 60% of the cases and can be used to exclude the possibility of intracranial arteriosclerosis – is so clear that it should be performed routinely before confirming the diagnosis by biopsy and beginning therapy.

Compared to angiography the benefit of MRI in the diagnosis of vasculitis is much more doubtful. The focal lesions in MRI are completely unspecific and do not correlate with the clinical symptoms. The significance of the small, pin-point-shaped lesions of high signal intensity in T2- and proton-density-weighted images seen in SLE patients is unclear [3]. MRI will probably be helpful for noninvasive follow-up of intracranial lesions and for monitoring therapy in these patients.

References

1. Albert DA, Rimon D, Silverstein MD (1989) Diagnosis of polyarteritis nodosa. I. A literature-based decision analysis approach. Radiology 171:886
2. Albert DA, Silverstein MD, Paunika K (1989) Diagnosis of polyarteritis nodosa. II. Empirical verification of a decision analysis model. Radiology 171:886
3. Berlit P, Röther J, Schwartz A, Bluestein HG (1992) Evaluation of cerebral disorders in systemic lupus erythematosus. Neurology 42 (Suppl 3):270
4. Borg M, Thomas P, Martin P (1989) Arterite cerebrale syphilitique. Evaluation therapeutique d'après les données angiographiques. Presse Med 18:1034
5. Bousser MG (1989) Les angietes du systeme nerveaux central. Rev Prat 39:2037–2040
6. Crouzet G, Agnettaz G, Pellat J, Perret J, Barge M (1974) Les voies de suppleance au cours du Moyamoya. J Neuroradiol 1:87–91
7. McAlindon TE, Ferguson IT (1989) Mononeuritis multiplex and occipital infarction complicating giant cell arteritis. Br J Rheumatol 28:257–258
8. McCormick WF, Schichet SS (1976). Atlas of cerebrovascular disease. Saunders, Philadelphia, pp 138–147
9. Salibi BS (1964) Bacteroid infection of the brain. Arch Neurol 10:629–634
10. Smith AS, Huang TE, Weinstein MA (1990) Periventricular involvement in CNS lymphomatoid granulomatosis: MR demonstration. J Comput Assist Tomogr 15:502–505
11. Stanson AW (1990) Roentgenographic findings in major vasculitic syndromes. Rheum Dis Clin North Am 16:293–308
12. Takayasu M (1908) Obliterative inflammatory alterations of the brachiocephalic arteries in a young female. Acta Soc Ophthalmol Jpn 12:554
13. Takeuchi K (1961) Occlusive disease of the carotid artery. Recent Adv Res Nerv Syst, Tokyo 5:511–514
14. Trevor RP, Sondheimer FK, Fessel WJ, Wolpert SM (1972) Angiographic demonstration of major vessel occlusion in systemic lupus erythematosus. Neuroradiology 4:202–205
15. Weiner DK, Allen NB (1991) Large vessel vasculitis of the central nervous system in systemic lupus erythematosus: report and review of the literature. J Rheumatol 18:748–751
16. Wylie EJ, Ehrenfeld WK (1970) Extracranial occlusive cerebrovascular disease: diagnosis and management. Saunders, Philadelphia Toronto London, pp 26–53

Giant Cell Arteritis

Peter Berlit and *Brigitte Storch-Hagenlocher*

1 Introduction

The two disorders included in the category of giant cell arteritis are temporal or cranial arteritis and Takayasu's arteritis, also called pulseless disease
or aortic arch arteritis. Both diseases are characterized histopathologically
by panarteritides of large or medium-sized arteries, with inflammatory
mononuclear cell infiltrates of the media, giant cell formation within vessel
walls, and destruction of the internal elastic lamina. Eventually, proliferation of intima leads to vessel occlusion.

The etiology and pathogenesis of giant cell arteritis remain unknown to
date, but discussion centers mainly on an immune pathogenesis. A genetic
predisposition and, possibly, infection seem to play a role, and most data
support a cell-mediated response against the vessel wall or its constituents
[4, 7, 28]. It is possible that the elastic membrane is the target of the
immunologic process. In temporal arteritis, the CD4 subset of lymphocytes
and macrophages dominate in the arterial lesions of the vessel wall [4, 41].
Deposition of circulating immune complexes, with subsequent activation of
the complement system, are of minor importance [20]. In Takayasu's arteritis it was observed that the majority of T cells were of the CD8 subset [29]. T
cells express HLA-DR antigens as part of immunologic activation. It is not
known whether activation is induced in situ or whether "homing" of activated T cells into the vessel wall occurs. A genetic predisposition in temporal arteritis is supported by its predominance in the white population, by the
familial aggregation, and by its association with HLA-DR antigens [6, 37,
44]. Takayasu's arteritis is rare in caucasians, but more frequent in oriental
populations. An HLA association is also observed in Takayasu's arteritis
[29].

2 Temporal Arteritis

In caucasians temporal arteritis is not a rare disease. The figures given for
the incidence in the USA and Europe mostly vary between 0.35 and 12.5 per
100000 [6, 7, 14, 15, 28, 31, 44], but several studies report the incidence in
the population over 50 years of age at about 18 per 100000 inhabitants. If

P. Berlit, P. M. Moore (Eds.)
Vasculitis, Rheumatic Disease
and the Nervous System
© Springer-Verlag Berlin Heidelberg 1993

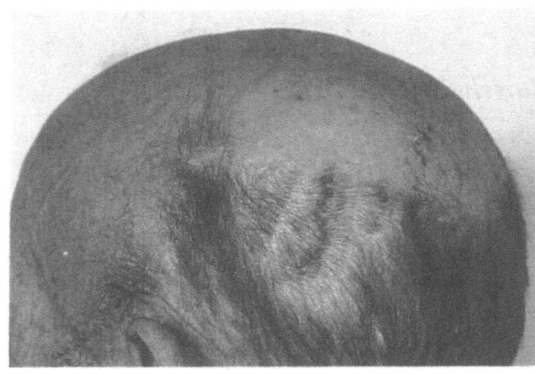

Fig. 1. Temporal arteritis: necrosis of the scalp

only histologically positive giant cell arteritis cases are considered, the average incidence is 5 cases per 100 000. Women are affected twice to three times as often as men. A doubling of the rate in women occurred in the 1980s while the rate in men remained stable [37, 44]. This observation has yet to be explained.

The average age at onset of temporal arteritis is between 67 and 72 years. The patients complain of persistent diffuse headaches, most prominent in the temporal area, and sometimes present with painful, swollen temporal arteries. Jaw claudication may occur. Atypically, but not rarely, pain occurs at the scalp, face, mouth, or tongue. Trophic disturbances cause localized hair loss and ulceration of the mucous membranes. Glossal necrosis and necrosis of the scalp due to involvement of the branches of the external carotid artery have been described [7, 9] (Fig. 1).

The classic inflammatory parameters in the serum are altered: there is usually a pronounced elevation of the erythrocyte sedimentation rate (ESR) and C-reactive protein is increased. In some cases histologically proven giant cell arteritis with normal ESR has been reported [47, 49]. The initial ESR is an important indicator of the prognosis of the disease [19]. Both exacerbations and complications are more frequent with an ESR greater than 90 mm in the first hour [7]. The patients often exhibit constitutional symptoms like fever, malaise, anorexia, and fatigue. Anemia is frequently present and may be hypochromic [11]. Acute phase reactants reflect the general inflammation. However, temporal arteritis can also present with the constitutional symptoms only. The frequency of this "silent presentation" is not known, but it is thought to be 10%–30% [21, 25].

The typical symptoms of temporal arteritis are frequently associated with muscle pain in the neck, shoulders, lower back, and the hips. Some authors consider temporal arteritis and polymyalgia rheumatica (PMR) to be one entity [3, 7, 14, 15]. The principal signs of PMR are symmetrical arthralgias and myalgias, particularly in the shoulder girdle, which is encountered in about 50% of patients with temporal arteritis.

The diagnosis of temporal arteritis is made on the basis of the clinical picture, ESR, age, and response to the administration of corticosteroids. To confirm the diagnosis, biopsy of the temporal artery is important. However, false-negative results may occur because of the segmental nature of the lesions [1]. Prompt biopsy is recommended, but typical histologic findings are sometimes obtained even 1 day after starting therapy [2, 24]. A segment of at least 2.5 cm in length should be taken. A combined histopathologic and immunohistologic examination of the biopsy material should be performed, since this increases the accuracy of the result [4, 32]. Where the symptoms and signs of temporal arteritis predominate, the temporal artery biopsy is positive more often than when the indicating symptoms are those of PMR. This holds true for both the pathologic and the immunohistochemical findings [32]. If the biopsy is negative on one side, biopsy material from the contralateral side or the occipital artery may be positive.

Major criteria for the diagnosis of temporal arteritis are:
– Age greater than 50 years
– Persistent headaches
– Symptoms of generalized disease (loss of weight, lack of appetite, fever, general feeling of illness)
– Initial ESR over 40 mm/h
– Morning stiffness of the larger joints
– Symmetrical arthralgias and myalgias in the pectoral or pelvic girdles
– Prompt response of the symptoms to corticosteroids

Complications of temporal arteritis include ophthalmologic, neurologic, visceral, and large artery disease.

The ocular complications of temporal arteritis have been best described. Visual problems range from transient blurring of vision to sudden and persistent blindness. Ocular involvement is found in 40% of untreated or insufficiently treated cases of temporal arteritis. The complication most feared is irreversible blindness, with a frequency of between 8% and 21% [7, 13, 18, 28]. Amaurosis may be caused by an ischemic lesion of the optic nerve because of involvement of the ciliary arteries, apoplexia papillae, or retrobulbar neuritis. Temporary visual disturbances such as transient monocular blindness, diplopia, and flimmer scotoma can precede blindness and must be taken as warning signs [30, 34]. Further ophthalmologic complications of giant cell arteritis are disturbances of pupillomotor response [40], ocular hypotonia, isolated ptosis [13], Horner's syndrome [5, 10], and visual field loss [35].

Cerebral ischemia is an occasional complication of temporal arteritis. The prevalence of this manifestation is generally considered to be about 10% [8, 13, 38]. Most frequently the posterior and middle cerebral arteries are affected. Among 50 patients studied at the Department of Neurology, Heidelberg, we saw a usually persistent central paresis in six patients. Vasculitis has been reported and confirmed by autopsy in the carotid arteries as well as in the vertebrobasilar circulation [8, 13, 22].

Temporal arteritis can also cause mental status abnormalities. This might be a chronic fluctuating delirium, delusional thinking, or memory impairment; sometimes concomitant symptoms of headache and visual loss are absent. Mental status abnormalities may also develop during treatment or drug tapering, and improve if steroids are raised [13]. A depressive syndrome at the onset of giant cell arteritis symptoms has been reported in up to 20% of patients [7].

Regarding the neurologic symptoms of temporal arteritis, Caselli et al. [13, 12] found a polyneuropathy or a mononeuropathy in 14% of 166 patients investigated with histologically proven temporal arteritis, a carpal tunnel syndrome being especially frequent [23]. Olfactory dysfunction and disturbances of the sense of taste have only rarely been reported with temporal arteritis [43]. We have seen it only in connection with Sjögren's syndrome [7].

Since giant cell arteritis is a generalized disease, circulatory disorders of the intestinal vessels [45], the coronary arteries [42], the renal arteries [46], the pulmonary arteries [16, 33], the breast [26], and the vessels of the uterus and adnexa [36] may occur. Takayasu's syndrome can be imitated by the giant cell arteritis of old age [39]. The prevalence of involvement of the aorta, subclavian artery, and the arteries of lower limbs is considered to be about 10%–15% [11, 15, 39, 42]. Symptoms are Raynaud's phenomenon, differences in blood pressure, abolition of the pulse, claudication of the limbs, muscle weakness, and paresthesia. Onset of these vascular manifestations is usually independent from the evolution of the classical symptoms, and they sometimes even occur several months after discontinuation of treatment. A careful physical examination may reveal visceral involvement early on. In addition to examining peripheral pulses and bilateral measurement of blood pressure, sonography is very helpful, especially of the aorta, the supraaortic vessels, and the arteries of the limbs.

The recurrence rate of temporal arteritis is high, the first year following diagnosis being particularly dangerous. Fundamentally, temporal arteritis is a nonfatal disease which has no influence on the statistical life expectancy of the patient, although in isolated cases it has been reported as the cause of death (myocardial infarction, aortic aneurysm, brain infarct) [3, 16, 42].

The treatment of choice for temporal arteritis is corticosteroids. There are no general recommendations for the dosage and the duration of corticosteroid therapy. Dosages of between 60 and 80 mg/day are recommended, daily administration being superior to the alternating form of therapy [27]. In general, the inital dose should be maintained over at least 3 weeks until, depending on the clinical symptoms and signs and ESR, it can be tapered by 5 mg/week to about 20 mg/day. Further reduction should not exceed a rate of 1 mg/month. The recommendations for length of therapy of temporal arteritis lie between 1 and 5 years. In a follow-up study of 49 patients, we found recurrence to be significantly more frequent with a period of treatment of less than 20 months [7], so in our experience a period of treatment of at least 2 years would seem appropriate. In long-term observation of the patient, and as a help in making a decision on the reduction or withdrawal of corticosteroid medication, determination of C-reactive protein should be taken into account in addition to measurement of the ESR [7]. A beneficial effect of azathioprine on reduction of steroid dosage has been described [17], but immunosuppressive drugs in general are not required in the treatment of temporal arteritis [15, 48].

3 Takayasu's Arteritis

Takayasu's arteritis predominantly affects women, but it is much less common than temporal arteritis, with an incidence rate of 2.6/1 million inhabitants. Takayasu's arteritis is more frequent in the Asiatic population. The diagnostic criteria for Takayasu's arteritis have been summarized by Ishikawa [29]:

Obligatory criterion: Age less than 40 years
Major criteria: Left mid subclavian lesion
                         Right mid subclavian lesion
Minor criteria: High ESR
                         Carotid artery tenderness
                         Hypertension
                         Pulmonary artery lesion
                         Left mid common carotid artery lesion
                         Distal brachiocephalic trunk lesion
                         Descending thoracic aorta lesion
                         Abdominal aorta lesion

In addition to the obligatory criterion, the presence of two major criteria, one major criterion and two or more minor criteria, or four or more minor criteria suggests a high probability of Takayasu's arteritis.

Neurologic complications of Takayasu's arteritis include headache, dizziness with syncopes, cerebral ischemia, and seizures. Trophic changes related to chronic hypoxia lead to lesions of the face and scalp, nose deformities and ocular symptoms. Death may occur because of congestive heart failure, mortality rates being reported at between 7% and 15% [29].

Besides the therapy of hypertension and congestive heart failure, steroids may be given in Takayasu's arteritis if the ESR is elevated. Suggested initial doses of prednisolone are 30–40 mg. In patients showing disease progression despite steroid treatment, cyclophosphamide or methotrexate (10–15 mg/week) may be tried. Steroid therapy at a dose of 7.5 mg/day should usually be continued for at least 2 years. In some patients surgical reconstruction of vessels becomes necessary. This holds true especially for patients with advanced obstructive vascular disease and normal ESR; in these cases steroids have no impact. On the other hand, surgery should not be performed in active disease until the inflammation is adequately controlled by steroids.

For both manifestations of giant cell arteritis, diagnosis rests on a high index of suspicion of the clinician, and the prognosis largely depends on the rapid performance of the appropriate diagnostic tests and consequent steroid treatment.

References

1. Albert DM, Hedges TR (1982) Significance of negative temporal artery biopsies. Trans Am Ophthalmol Soc 80:143–154
2. Allison MC, Gallagher PJ (1984) Temporal artery biopsy and corticosteroid treatment. Ann Rheum Dis 43:416–417
3. Andersson R, Malmvall BE, Bengtsson BA (1986) Long-term survival in giant cell arteritis including temporal arteritis and polymyalgia rheumatica. Acta Med Scand 220:361–364
4. Banks PM, Cohen MD, Ginsburg WW, Hunder GG (1983) Immunohistologic and cytochemical studies of temporal arteritis. Arthritis Rheum 26:1201–1207
5. Bell TAG, Gibson RA, Tullo AB (1980) A case of giant cell arteritis and Horner's syndrome. Scand Med J 25:302
6. Bengtsson BA, Malmvall BE (1981) The epidemiology of giant cell arteritis including temporal arteritis and polymyalgia rheumatica. Arthritis Rheum 7:899–904
7. Berlit P (1992) Clinical and laboratory findings with giant-cell-arteritis. J Neurol Sci 111:1–12
8. Bogousslavsky J, Deruaz JP, Regli F (1985) Bilateral obstruction of internal carotid artery from giant cell arteritis and massive infarction limited to the vertebrobasilar area. Eur Neurol 24:57–61
9. Bowlder DA, Knight JR (1985) Lingual claudication and necrosis as a complication of giant cell arteritis. J Laryngol Otol 99:417–420
10. Bromfield EB, Slakter JS (1988) Horner's yndrome in temporal arteritis. Arch Neurol 45:604
11. Calamia KT, Hunder GG (1980) Clinical manifestations of giant cell (temporal) arteritis. Clin Rheum Dis 6:389–403
12. Caselli RJ, Hunder GG, Whisnant JP (1988) Neurologic disease in biopsy-proven giant cell (temporal) arteritis. Neurology 38:352–359
13. Caselli RJ, Daube JR, Hunder GG, Whisnant JP (1988) Peripheral neuropathic syndromes in giant cell (temporal) arteritis. Neurology 38:685–689
14. Chuang TY, Hunder GG, Duane M, Ilstrup MS Kurland L (1982) Polymyalgia rheumatica. A 10-year epidemiologic and clinical study. Ann Int Med 97:672–680
15. Delecoeuillerie G, Joly P, Cohen de Lara A, Paolaggi JB (1988) Polymyalgia rheumatica and temporal arteritis: a retrospective analysis of prognostic features and different corticosteroid regimens (11 year survey of 210 patients). Ann Rheum Dis 47:733–739
16. Dennison AR, Watkins RM, Gunning AJ (1985) Simultaneous aortic and pulmonary artery aneurysms due to giant cell arteritis. Thorax 40:156–157
17. De Silva M, Hazleman BL (1986) Azathioprine in giant cell arteritis/polymyalgia rheumatica: a double-blind study. Ann Rheum Dis 45:136–138
18. Dutoit A, Dubus V, Croccel L, Routier G, Godeau P (1988) Clinical and developmental aspects of Horton's disease. Retrospective study of 100 cases. Ann Cardiol Angiol (Paris) 37:199–204
19. Ellis MS, Ralston S (1983) The ESR in the diagnosis and management of the polymyalgia rheumatica/giant cell arteritis syndromes. Ann Rheum Dis 42:168–170
20. Espinoza LR, Bridgeford P, Lowenstein M (1982) Polymyalgia rheumatica and giant cell arteritis: circulating immune complexes. J Rheumatol 9:556–560
21. Gallagher CG, Gallagher E, Crowe JP (1985) Asymptomatic giant cell arteritis. Arch Intern Med 145:2122

22. Gibb WR, Urry PA, Lees AJ (1985) Giant cell arteritis with spinal cord infarction and basilar artery thrombosis. J Neurol Neurosurg Psychiatry 48:945–948
23. Golbus J, McCune JW (1987) Giant cell arteritis and peripheral neuropathy: a report of 2 cases and review of literature. J Rheumatol 14:129–134
24. Hall S, Lie JT, Kurland LT, Persellin S, O'Brien PC, Hunder GG (1983) The therapeutic impact of temporal artery biopsy. Lancet 2:1217–1220
25. Healey LA Wilske KR (1980) Presentation of occult giant cell arteritis. Arthritis Rheum 23:641–644
26. Horne D, Crabtree TS, Lewkonia RM (1987) Breast arteritis in polymyalgia rheumatica. J Rheumatol 14:613–615
27. Hunder GG, Sheps SG, Allen GL, Joyce JW (1975) Daily and alternate-day corticosteroid regiments in treatment of giant cell arteritis. Ann Int Med 82:613–618
28. Huston KA, Hunder GG, Lie JT, Kennedy RH, Eiverback LA (1978) Temporal arteritis: a 25-year epidemiologic, clinical and pathologic study. Ann Int Med 88:162–167
29. Ishikawa K (1978) Natural history and classification of occlusive thromboaortopathy (Takayasu's disease). Circulation 57:28–39
30. Jay WM, Nazarian SM (1986) Bilateral sixth nerve pareses with temporal arteritis and diabetes. J Clin Neuroophthalmol 6:91–95
31. Jonasson F, Cullen KF, Elton RA (1979) Temporal arteritis: a 14-year epidemiological, clinical and prognostic study. Scot Med J 24:111–117
32. Knecht S, Henningsen H, Rauterberg EW, Berlit P (1989) Immunhistologische Untersuchungen zur Polymyalgia rheumatica und Arteriitis temporalis. Verh Dtsch Ges Neurol 5:626–628
33. Kramer MR, Melzer E, Nesher G, Sonnenblick M (1987) Pulmonary manifestations of temporal arteritis. Eur J Respir Dis 71:430–433
34. Lipton RB, Solomon S, Wertenbaker C (1985) Gradual loss and recovery of vision in temporal arteritis. Arch Intern Med 145:2252–2253
35. Lipton RB, Rosenbaum D, Mehler MF (1987) Giant cell arteritis causes recurrent posterior circulation transient ischemic attacks which respond to corticosteroids. Eur Neurol 27:97–100
36. Lui IOL, Taylor W, Chin SH (1985) Giant cell arteritis of the uterus and adnexa: case report. Br J Obstet Gynaecol 92:1064
37. Machado EBV, Michet CJ, Ballard DJ, Hunder GG, Beard CM, Chu CP, O'Fallon WM (1988) Trends in incidence and clinical presentation of temporal arteritis in Olmsted Country, Minnesota, 1950–1985. Arthritis Rheum 31:745–749
38. Michotte A, de Keyser J, Dierckx R, Impens N, Solheid C, Ebinger G (1986) Brain stem infarction as a complication of giant cell arteritis. Clin Neurol Neurosurg 88:127–129
39. Perruquet JL, Davis DE, Harrington TM (1986) Aortic arch arteritis in the elderly. Arch Int Med 146:289–291
40. Rabinowich L, Mehler MF (1988) Parasympathetic pupillary involvement in biopsy-proven temporal arteritis. Ann Ophthalmol 20:400–402
41. Robb-Nicholson C, Chang RW, Anderson S, Roberts WN, Green J, Longtime J, Corson J, Larson M, George D, Bryant G, Liang MH (1988) Diagnostic value of the history and examination in giant cell arteritis: a clinical pathological study of 81 artery biopsies. J Rheumatol 15:1793–1796
42. Säve-Söderbergh J, Malmvall BO, Andersson R, Bengtsson BA (1986) Giant cell arteritis as a cause of death. Report of nine cases. JAMA 255:493–496
43. Schon F (1988) Involvement of smell and taste in giant cell arteritis. J Neurol Neurosurg Psychiatry 51:1594
44. Smith CA, Fidler WJ, Pinals RS (1983) The epidemiology of giant cell arteritis. Report of a ten-year study in Shelby County, Tennessee. Arthritis Rheum 26:1214–1219
45. Smith JA, O'Sullivan M, Gough J, Williams BD (1988) Small-intestinal perforation secondary to localized giant cell arteritis of the mesenteric vessels. Br J Rheumatol 27:236–238

46. Truong L, Kopelman RG, Williams GS, Pirani CL (1985) Temporal arteritis and renal disease. Case report and review of literature. Am J Med 78:171–175
47. Villalta J, Estrach T (1985) Temporal arteritis with normal sedimentation rate. Ann Int Med 103:808
48. Wendling D, Hory B, Blanc D (1985) Cyclosporine: a new adjuvant therapy for giant cell arteritis? Arthritis Rheum 28:1078–1079
49. Wong RL, Korn JH (1986) Temporal arteritis without an elevated sedimentation rate. Case report and review of the literature. Am J Med 80:959–964

Granulomatous Vasculitides: Neurologic Aspects

Wolfgang L. Gross, Andreas C. Arlt, and Wilhelm H. Schmitt

1 Introduction

The term "systemic vasculitis" is used to describe a variety of syndromes or diseases characterized pathologically by inflammation of the blood vessels and clinically by: (a) the consequences of vascular lesion (e.g., occlusion leading to infarction); (b) constitutional symptoms (e.g., fever, weight loss, night sweating); and (c) "uncharacteristic" rheumatic complaints (e.g., arthralgia, myalgia, frank arthritis).

In patients with systemic vasculitis, neurologic problems frequently lead to various clinical symptoms, and peripheral and – less often – CNS manifestations occur. These arise most frequently in the polyarteritis nodosa group and in rheumatoid vasculitis [17, 27, 28, 38, 39]. Furthermore, in many cases, vasculitic neuropathy is the initial manifestation of systemic vasculitis, heralding the onset of systemic disease [28]. Finally, neuropathy may be the sole manifestation of vasculitis [17]. Various diagnostic, prognostic, and therapeutic problems are thus associated with vasculitis.

2 Classification

By definition, the cause (or causes) of primary or idiopathic vasculitis are unknown. Secondary vasculitis can be due to primary diseases such as infections, connective tissue diseases, chronic granulomatous disorders – sarcoidosis and Crohn's disease – malignancies, and drug reactions and abuse. The secondary vasculitides may resemble the classical idiopathic forms, both clinically and morphologically. Consequently, underlying causes of vasculitis must be rigorously excluded. For the purposes of classification the various types of idiopathic (or primary) vasculitis are grouped according to the size of the affected vessels and the form of histologic infiltrate (granulomatous and non-granulomatous arteritides) (Table 1).

This article reviews only two granulomatous vasculitides: Wegener's granulomatosis (WG) and Churg–Strauss syndrome (CSS), since the giant cell arteritides do not usually form true granulomata (for review see [3]). They are vasculitides with giant cells in the vessel wall (e.g., temporal arteritis and Takayasu's arteritis; see Berlit and Storch-Hagenlocher, this volume,

P. Berlit, P. M. Moore (Eds.)
Vasculitis, Rheumatic Disease
and the Nervous System
© Springer-Verlag Berlin Heidelberg 1993

Table 1. Classification of primary vasculitis

Vessel type	Granuloma +	Granuloma –
Large	Giant cell arteritis	
Medium	Churg–Strauss syndrome	Classic polyarteritis
Small	Wegener's granulomatosis	Microscopic polyarteritis

pp. 33). Lymphomatoid granulomatosis is not considered here because it may be included in the neoplastic (malignant) lymphoma group. This review focuses on current pathodynamic aspects in both diseases. It presents the new classification criteria given by the American College of Rheumatology (ACR) in 1990, and introduces a new immunopathogenic working hypothesis based on the ANCA (antineutrophilic cytoplasmic autoantibody) findings. It delineates diagnostic and treatment strategies and reports typical neurologic problems seen in a clinic for rheumatic diseases.

3 Wegener's Granulomatosis

WG was first described by Klinger and then recognized as a disease entity by Wegener in 1936 (for review see [50]). WG is a primary vasculitis characterized by the presence of a necrotizing granulomatous vasculitis of the upper and lower respiratory tract associated with a necrotizing glomerulonephritis [49]. Because up until 1985 laboratory findings were nonspecific, the diagnosis was usually based on the combination of typical clinical features and compatible histopathology. Consequently, WG was recognized and treated only when the disease was in a "full blown" state. However, in 1966, Carrington and Liebow described a particular from of WG associated with similar histologic features but limited to the lungs [5]. Since then, the presence of the complete syndrome consisting of "Wegener's triad" [21] has not been regarded as necessary for diagnosis. There is clinical and histopathologic evidence for the disease having a two-phase course (Fig. 1): The classic syndrome represents the later, generalized phase of a disease process characterized by symptoms of variable duration limited to the upper and/or lower respiratory tract [4, 22, 23, 46]. The criteria for classification of WG set up by the American College of Rheumatology (ACR) in 1990 recognize the variable aspects of clinical presentation (Table 2).

In most instances the nose, ear and throat are affected first (Friedrich Wegener: "rhinogenic granulomatosis"; for review see [22, 41]). The earliest nasal manifestation is obstruction due to mucosal swelling, but most patients present with a more advanced stage characterized by nasal bleeding and intra- or external nasal deformity. A serosanguineous discharge is common. Granulations and septal perforation often occur. Saddling of the nose is a common finding (about 10%). Approximately half the cases with nasal involvement also have paranasal sinus involvement.

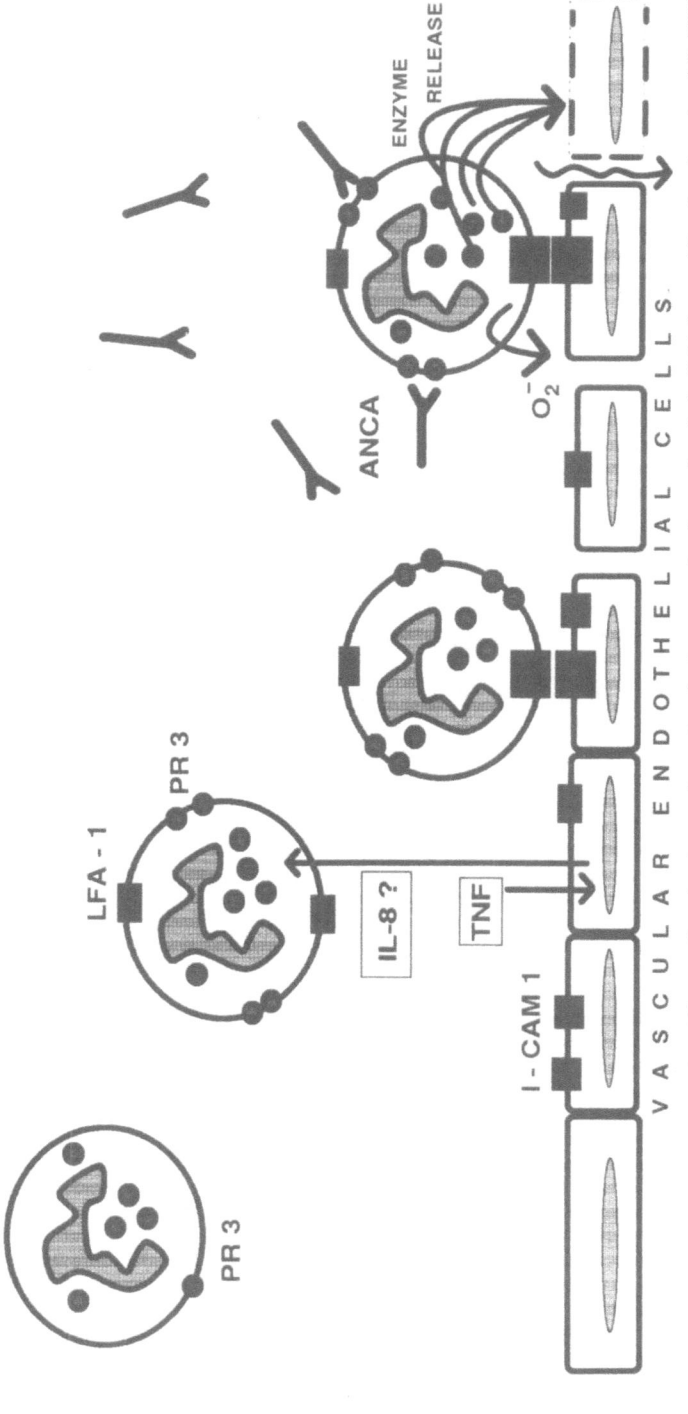

Fig. 1a–c. Hypothetical model of ANCA-mediated polymorphonuclear leukocyte activation and endothelial injury. **a** Unprimed neutrophil; PR3 mostly sequestered in azurophil granules. **b** Priming of neutrophils by cytokines; intracytoplasmic PR3 is translocated to the cell surface and becomes accessible to ANCA. **c** Interaction between ANCA and antigen leads to activation of the neutrophils, with degranulation, generation of oxygen radicals, and endothelial cell injury. (Modified from [26])

Table 2. The American College of Rheumatology 1990 criteria for the classification of Wegener's granulomatosis

Criterion	Definition
1. Nasal or oral inflammation	Development of painful or painless oral ulcers or purulent or bloody nasal discharge
2. Abnormal chest radiograph	Chest radiograph showing the presence of nodules, fixed infiltrates, or cavities
3. Urinary sediment	Microhematuria (> 5 red cells per high power field) or red cell casts in urine sediment
4. Granulomatous inflammation	Histologic changes showing granulomatous inflammation within the wall of an artery or in the perivascular or extravascular area (artery or arteriole)

For purposes of classification, a patient shall be said to have WG if at least two of four criteria are met (sensitivity 88.2%, specificity 92.0%).

A definitive diagnosis on the basis of a nasal biopsy is rare. Biopsy specimens from the affected paranasal sinus reveal better results. and so we and others prefer to confirm the diagnosis histologically by a biopsy from the ear–nose–throat region; open lung biopsy is much more agressive [15, 34, 42].

Clinically, the primary nasal lesion spreads by continuous growth, resulting in otologic manifestations in the middle, inner, and external ear. This can lead to polychondritis of the ear, to serous and sometimes suppurative otitis media, and to sensorineural deafness and vertigo due to involvement of the former. Furthermore, the granulomatous process can cause nasolacrimal duct obstruction and proptosis (due to retroorbital granulomatous masses), invasion of the intracranium, and involvement of the oral cavity, oropharynx, and larynx. The neurologic effects are listed in Table 3.

Table 3. Neurologic involvement (modified from [41])

Extent of disease			
Limited		**Systemic**	
CNS	PNS	CNS	PNS
Granuloma at skull base	Cranial nerve involvement	Thrombosis	Polyneuropathy
		Hemorrhage	Mononeuropathy multiplex
Diabetes insipidus	Proptosis		
Meningitis			

Initially, the clinical manifestations are not life-threatening. However, ulcerative lesions or an inflammatory pseudotumor in the subglottic region may cause respiratory distress. Less frequently, bronchial stenoses may cause atelectasis, lobar collapse, or obstructive pneumonia. Nodular infiltrates, which may cavitate, are typical lung findings. Microscopically, the lesions show a necrotizing granulomatous vasculitis with an infiltrate of neutrophils, lymphocytes, plasma cells, histiocytes, and giant cells.

Neurologic manifestations may be due to local complications of the granulomatous process or systemic vasculitis. The underlying pathogenic process in the CNS or cranial nerve involvement is difficult to evaluate. In most cases a combination of clinical and neurophysiologic examinations, cerebrospinal fluid analysis, computed tomography (CT), and magnetic resonance imaging (MRI) lead to a useful diagnosis. Immunohistochemical studies of pulmonary tissue have revealed that the lymphoid infiltrates are predominantly T cells and monocytes. Thus, in several centers open thoracotomy and lung biopsy are recommended to establish the diagnosis [34]. Since these limited forms of WG are being recognized increasingly early, it has become clear that they have a subacute or chronic course of unpredictable duration before they turn into the generalized phase characterized by systemic vasculitis, usually with renal involvement.

As mentioned above, peripheral neuropathy may herald the onset and course of the systemic process. About 50% of WG patients manifest a peripheral neuropathy which typically improves. The peripheral neuropathy associated with systemic vasculitis has a good prognosis in terms of functional neurologic recovery [6, 17, 28, 40] and has little effect on survival rate. It is, however, an indicator of a vasculitic process [28].

Rheumatic complaints, constitutional symptoms, and frank vasculitic lesions (for example episcleritis – "red eye" – or purpura of the skin) are frequently ominous signs heralding the systemic disease. Thus, the capillaritis can lead to the pulmonary–renal syndrome characterized by alveolar hemorrhage and rapidly progressive glomerulonephritis. Cardiac involvement often occurs with acute generalized WG; however, severe granulomatous giant cell myocarditis leading to fatal complications [51] is, in contrast to CSS, rather infrequent.

Attempts have been made to find a classification of disease extent and severity which would allow prognostic statements or facilitate therapeutic decisions. The "ELK classification" (Table 4) of DeRemee and Specks has proved to be useful for clinical practice [46]. To take into account the two-phase course of the disease and to emphasize the dangerous systemic phase of WG we have extended this classification [23, 42].

According to these pathodynamic events, neurologic problems are phase-dependent. Partly due to diagnostic problems, CNS manifestations are, or appear to be, infrequent and follow-up is difficult. In a recent preliminary study, MRI scans were slightly superior to CT scans in the detecting of CNS vasculitis [29]. However, peripheral nervous system involvement is more common and probably an early sign of systemic spread of the disease.

Table 4. Extended "ELK classification" of Wegener's granulomatosis: frequency of symptoms in 186 patients with generalized WG (modified from [24])

Code	Symptom	Frequency (%)
E	Ear, nose, throat	80
L	Lung	59
K	Kidney	81
A	Rheumatic complaints	57
P	Peripheral nervous system	50
C	Central nervous system	21
B	Constitutional symptoms	22
Ey	Eye	38
H	Heart	9
G	Gastrointestinal tract	17
S	Skin	21

Accurate neurophysiologic investigation provides valuable data for assessing disease activity [28].

Antineutrophilic cytoplasmic autoantibodies (ANCAs) specific for constituents of neutrophil primary granules and monocyte lysosomes have been demonstrated in vasculitic disorders since 1982 (for review see [24, 31]). Using indirect immunofluorescence technique on alcohol-fixed granulocytes, three different staining patterns allow the distinction among three types of ANCA:

1. Classic antineutrophilic cytoplasmic antibody (cANCA, formerly known as ACPA)
2. An artificial perinuclear/nuclear staining pattern (pANCA)
3. A mixture of c- and pANCA (xANCA, also recently subsumed under pANCA)

When aldehyde- instead of alcohol-fixed neutrophils are used, c- and pANCA cannot be discriminated and both appear as the same pure cytoplasmic staining pattern. Most cANCA are directed against proteinase 3 (PR3, "Wegener's autoantigen"). cANCA are found in the sera of at least 90% of generalized and 50% of initial phase WG patients but not in a wide spectrum of diseases other than WG. However, cANCA have been sporadically described in sera from polyarteritis (mostly the microscopic form) and CSS patients. In most cases of WG, cANCA titers correlate with clinical activity and become negative during complete remission [11, 42].

On the other hand, the pANCA fluorescence is mostly induced by anti-myeloperoxidase antibodies and to a smaller extent by others (targets known include elastase, cathepsin G, lactoferrin). Some pANCAs specific for myeloperoxidase are associated with idiopathic crescentic glomerulonephritis, microscopic polyarteritis, and other systemic vasculitides exhibiting only pauci-immune deposits in the walls of blood vessels. pANCA fluorescence is rarely found in WG ($<$ 10%) and appears to be slightly more frequent in CSS [12, 31].

In addition to their diagnostic usefulness as serologic markers, ANCAs may be directly involved in the pathogenesis of systemic vasculitis [26, 32]. We have shown that PR3, a lysosomal protein localized in the azurophilic granula, is expressed on the cell surface of normal neutrophils. Thus, the antigen is accessible for circulating anti-PR3 antibodies [13], a prerequisite for their postulated pathogenetic significance. Subsequently, it has been shown that ANCAs are able to activate cytokine-primed granulocytes and monocytes to undergo a respiratory burst and degranulation [31].

This effect is of special importance under the conditions of a "hypercyto-kinemia" (high levels of tumor necrosis factor and other mediators of inflammation). Here, the expression of adhesion molecules on both vascular endothelial cells (intercellular adhesion molecule 1, ICAM-1; endothe-lial–leukocyte adhesion factor 1, E-LAM-1) and primed neutrophils (lym-phocyte function associated antigen 1, LFA-1) results in a close "physical" relation between both cell types. Thus, the release of oxygen radicals and lysosomal enzymes becomes especially harmful to the endothelial monolayer of the vessels involved, resulting in necrotizing vasculitis (Fig. 1). This hypothesis is supported by the recent finding that ANCA-activated granulo-cytes are able to injure endothelial cells in vitro [18].

Beside ANCA, T cells may well be important for the pathogenesis of WG. The occurrence of granuloma and the renal (glomerular) T-cell infiltra-tion suggest an autoreactive T-cell response. It has been shown that lympho-cytes from WG patients proliferate when exposed to PR3 in vitro (Mayet, personal communication). Furthermore, the soluble interleukin-2 receptor – a marker of T-cell activation – correlates well with disease activity [43]. Thus, both T- and B-cell mechanisms seem to be involved in the pathogene-sis of WG.

In conclusion, the diagnosis of WG is based on clinical symptoms and histology. Because cANCA (anti-PR3 autoantibodies) are strongly asso-ciated with WG (specificity about 90%) they are an important seromarker for this disease.

4 Churg–Strauss Syndrome

Jacob Churg and Lotte Strauss first described a disease known as "allergic granulomatosis and angiitis" or simply by the eponym "Churg–Strauss syn-drome (CSS)" (for review see [1, 40]). They described a group of patients with asthma, peripheral eosinophilia, and systemic vasculitis. There is a considerable overlap between several entities in the idiopathic systemic vasculitis group and CSS, e.g., the combination CSS plus temporal arteritis [2], WG [30], and others (see [36]). CSS closely resembles Kussmaul–Maier polyarteritis nodosa [36]; however, there are characteristic features that distinguish this syndrome as a distinct entity. There are also a number of clinical and pathologic features of WG, which therefore needs to be considered in the differential diagnosis.

In contrast to classic polyarteritis nodoas, pulmonary involvement (commonly asthma) is seen in virtually all CSS patients, and even severe alveolar hemorrhage and/or pulmonary–renal syndrome may develop [9]. Peripheral (blood) eosinophilia, eosinophilic tissue infiltrates, and eosinophilia in the bronchoalveolar lavage can be detected. Vasculitis can affect small vessels in addition to medium-sized arteries. Granulomatous lesions are common and can be found in vascular and extravascular locations. Glomerulonephritis is only seen in a minority of cases and rarely as a rapidly progressive form. However, as in all other vasculitides, the clinical spectrum of CSS varies considerably from the perspectives of the different medical disciplines. For example, according to nephrologists, glomerulonephritis is not as rare as commonly thought [10, 33].

More recently (1977), DeRemee's group worked out three phases of the disease. A prodromal phase, which may persist for years, is characterized by allergic reactions such as allergic rhinitis, nasal polyposis, and at a later stage bronchial asthma. In the second phase peripheral blood and tissue eosinophilia can be detected. Clinically, Löffler's syndrome, chronic eosinophilic pneumonia, or even eosinophilic gastroenteritis may occur. The eosinophilic infiltrates may recur over years before the third phase, consisting of a life-threatening systemic vasculitis, is reached. Again, it must be stressed that, as in WG, not all cases proceed from a limited to a generalized stage and some patients initially present a severe vasculitic disease.

The etiopathogenetic aspects of CSS cannot be presented in detail in the present paper. Because the clinical and pathologic features of CSS can be mimicked by parasitic infections [7] or eosinophilia–myalgia syndrome due to ingestion of l-tryptophan [48], a "secondary" form of vasculitis must be excluded. More recently a detailed differential diagnosis between CSS and allergic fungal sinusitis has also been published [45].

Although chest X-ray findings in CSS can be similar to those of WG, the pulmonary lesions in allergic angiitis and granulomatosis rarely cavitate. In full-blown disease, the clinical picture is similar to that seen in classic polyarteritis, with the exception of pulmonary involvement. The cutaneous lesions usually include purpura and nodules – from which a histologic diagnosis can be made – but a variety of other lesions have been observed [20].

Whereas renal and lung involvement appear to be negative prognostic factors in WG, most deaths in CSS are due to cardiac involvement, which occurs in about 40% of cases. As in classic polyarteritis nodosa and WG, peripheral nerve involvement is a common aspect of CSS, especially when the disease is already advanced. Asthma often precedes the onset of neuropathic symptoms by months or even years [28]. Neuropathy has occurred in about two thirds of the cases reported so far. The typical lesion is mononeuritis multiplex, but in some patients an asymmetrical or symmetrical peripheral neuropathy is seen. Cranial nerve palsies are infrequent; the most common cranial nerve lesion is an ischemic optic neuritis. Although

Churg and Strauss reported that 8 of their 13 patients had CNS manifestations, there is an overall prevalence of about 27% in the more recent literature. Nevertheless, cerebral hemorrhage/infarction is a major cause of morbidity and death in patients with CSS.

5 Treatment

Before the introduction of immunosuppressive therapy, the course of WG was uniformly fatal (for review see [50]). In contrast, CSS has been regarded as less dangerous than WG. However, with the experience gained from larger numbers of patients one has to accept that there is neither a uniform course of WG nor is CSS always a more benign disease [46].

The limited form of WG (initial phase) responds to cotrimoxazole and/or to prednisone [16, 47]. By contrast, the treatment of choice in the generalized form is a combined therapy with corticosteroids and cyclophosphamide (Fauci regimen) [19]. Severe cases respond best to the Fauci regimen; less severe cases can be treated less aggressively by bolus cyclophosphamide [14, 47].

CSS usually responds well to corticosteroids. However, more severe cases with cardiac problems should be treated by the Fauci regimen or by cyclophosphamide bolus therapy [8].

References

1. Alarcsn-Segovia, D (1990) Polyarteritis nodosa, Churg–Strauss syndrome, and other eosinophilic syndromes. Curr Opin Rheumatol 2:50
2. Amato MBP, Barbas CSV, Delmonte VC, Carvalho CRR (1988) Concurrent Churg-Strauss syndrome and temporal arteritis in a young patient with pulmonary nodules. Am Rev Respir Dis 139:1539–1542
3. Bengtsson BA, Andersson R (1991) Giant cell and Takayasu's arteritis. Curr Opin Rheumatol 3:1
4. Boudes P (1990) Purely granulomatous Wegener's granulomatosis: a new concept for an old disease. Sem Arthritis Rheum 19:365–370
5. Carrington CB et al. (1969) Chronic eosinophilic pneumonia. New Engl J Med 280:787–798
6. Chang RW, Bell CL, Hallett M (1984) Clinical characteristics and prognosis of vasculitic mononeuropathy multiplex. Arch Neurol 41:618–621
7. Chauhan A, Scott DGI, Neuberger J, Gaston JSH, Bacon PA (1990) Churg–Strauss vasculitis and ascaris infection. Ann Rheum Dis 49:320–3228
8. Chow CC, Li EKM, Lai FM (1989) Allergic granulomatosis and angiitis (Churg-Strauss syndrome): response to "pulse" intravenous cyclophosphamide. Ann Rheum Dis 48:605–608
9. Clutterbuck EJ, Pusey CD (1987) Severe alveolar haemorrhage in Churg–Strauss syndrome. Eur J Respir Dis 71:158–163
10. Clutterbuck EJ, Evans DJ, Pusey CD (1990) Renal involvement in Churg–Strauss syndrome. Nephrol Dial Transplant 5:161–167
11. Cohen Tervaert JW, van der Woude FJ, Fauci AS, Ambrus JL, Velosa J, Keane WF, Meijer S, van der Giessen M, The TH, van der Hem GK, Kallenberg CGM (1989) Association between active Wegener's granulomatosis and anticytoplasmic antibodies. Arch Intern Med 149:2461–2465

12. Cohen Tervaert JW, Goldschmeding R, Elema JD, Limburg PC, van der Giessen M, Huitema MG, Koolen MI, Heni RJ, The TH, van der Hem GK, von dem Borne AEGK, Kallenberg CGM (1990) Association of autoantibodies to myeloperoxidase with different forms of vasculitis. Arthritis Rheum 33:1264–1272

13. Csernok E, Lüdemann J, Gross WL, Bainton DF (1990) Ultrastructural localisation of proteinase 3, the target antigen of anti-cytoplasmic antibodies circulating in Wegener's granulomatosis. Am J Pathol 137:1113–1120

14. Cupps TR (1990) Cyclophosphamide: to pulse or not to pulse? Am J Med 89:399–402

15. DelBuono EA, Flint A (1991) Diagnostic usefulness of nasal biopsy in Wegener's granulomatosis. Human Pathol 22:107–110

16. DeRemee RA (1988) The treatment of Wegener's granulomatosis with trimethoprim sulfamethoxazole: illusion or vision? Arthritis Rheum 31:31

17. Dyck PJ, Benstead TJ, Conn DL, Stevens JC, Windebank AJ, Low PA (1987) Nonsystemic vasculitic neuropathy. Brain 110:843–853

18. Ewert B, Falk RJ, Jennette JC (1990) Anti-neutrophil cytoplasmic antibodies stimulate neutrophils to injure endothelial monolayers in vitro (abstract). Third international workshop on ANCA, Washington

19. Fauci AS, Haynes BF, Katz P, Wolff SM (1983) Wegener's granulomatosis: prospective clinical and therapeutic experience with 85 patients for 21 years. Ann Intern Med:98:76–85

20. Gibson LE (1990) Granulomatous vasculitides and the skin. Dermatol Clinics 8:335–345

21. Godman GC, Churg J (1954) Wegener's granulomatosis. AMA Arch Path 58:533

22. Gross WL (1989) Wegener's granulomatosis. New aspects of the disease course, immunodiagnostic procedures and stage-adapted treatment. Sarcoidosis 6:15

23. Gross WL, Lüdemann G, Kiefer G, Lehmann H (1986) Anticytoplasmic antibodies in Wegener's granulomatosis. Lancet i:809

24. Gross WL, Lüdemann J, Csernok E (1990) Autoantibodies ANCA/ACPA in vasculitis: history, nomenclature, target antigens, clinical impact, and pathogenesis. Clin Immunol Newsletter 10:159–163

25. Gross WL, Schmitt WH, Csernok E (1991) Anti-neutrophil cytoplasmic antibody associated diseases: a rheumatologist's perspective. Am J Kidney Dis 18:175–179

26. Gross WL, Csernok E, Schmitt WH (1991) Anti-neutrophil cytoplasmic antibodies: immunobiological aspects. Klin Wochenschr 69:558–566

27. Guillevin L, Du LTH, Godeau P, Jais P, Wechsler B (1988) Clinical findings of prognosis of polyarteritis nodosa and Churg–Strauss angiitis: a study in 165 patients. Br J Rheumatol 27:258–264

28. Hawke SHB, Davies L, Pamphlett R, Guo YP, Pollard JD, McLeod JG (1991) Vasculitic neuropathy. A clinical and pathological study. Brain 114:2175–2190

29. Hellmann DB, Roubenhoff R, Healy RA, Wong H (1991) Central nervous system vasculitis: comparison of central nervous system angiography with computerized tomography and magnetic resonance (abstract). Arthritis Rheum 34 (Suppl 9):S73

30. Henochowicz S, Eggensperger D, Pierce L, Barth WF (1986) Necrotizing systemic vasculitis with features of both Wegener's granulomatosis and Churg–Strauss vasculitis. Arthritis Rheum 29:565–569

31. Jennette JC, Falk RJ (1990) Antineutrophil cytoplasmic autoantibodies and associated diseases: a review. Am J Kidney 6:517–529

32. Kallenberg CGM, Cohen Tervaert JW, van der Woude FJ, Goldschmeding R, von dem Borne AEGK, Weening JJ (1991) Autoimmunity to lysosomal enzymes: new clues to vasculitis and glomerulonephritis? Immunol Today 12:61–64

33. Lanham JG, Elkon KB, Pusey CD, Hughes GR (1984) Systemic vasculitis with asthma and eosinophilia: a clinical approach to the Churg–Strauss syndrome. Medicine 63:65–81

34. Leavitt RY, Fauci AS (1990) Wegener's granulomatosis and other systemic granulomatous conditions. Curr Opin Rheumatol 2:55–59

35. Leavitt RY, Fauci AS, Bloch DA, Michel BA, Hunder GG, Arend WP, Calabrese LH, Fries JF, Lie JT, Lightfoot RW Jr, Masi AT, McShane DJ, Mills JA, Stevens MB, Wallace SL, Zvaifler NJ (1990) Criteria for the classification of Wegener's granulomatosis. American College of Rheumatology. Arthritis Rheum 33:1101–1106
36. Lightfoot RW Jr (1991) Churg–Strauss syndrome and polyarteritis nodosa. Curr Opin Rheumatol 3:1–16
37. Masi AT, Hunder GG, Lie JT, Michel BA, Bloch DA, Arend WP, Calabrese LH, Edworthy SM, Fauci AS, Leavitt RY, Lightfoot RW Jr, McShane DJ, Mills JA, Stevens MB, Wallace SL, Zvaifler NJ (1990) Criteria for the classification of Churg-Strauss syndrome (allergic granulomatosis and angiitis). American College of Rheumatology. Arthritis Rheum 33:1094–1098
38. McCombe PA, McLeod JG, Pollard JD, Guo YP, Ingall TJ (1987) Peripheral sensorimotor and autonomic neuropathy associated with systemic lupus erythematosus: clinical, pathological and immunological features. Brain 110:533–549
39. Moore PM, Cupps TR (1983) Neurological complications of vasculitis. Ann Neurol 14:155–167
40. Moore PM, Fauci AS (1981) Neurologic manifestations of systemic vasculitis: a retrospective and prospective study of the clinicopathologic features and responses to therapy in 25 patients. Am J Med 71:517–524
41. Murty GE (1990) Wegener's granulomatosis: otorhinolaryngological manifestations. Clin Otolaryngol 15:385–393
42. Nölle B, Specks U, Lüdemann J, Rohrbach MS, DeRemee RA, Gross WL (1989) Anticytoplasmatic autoantibodies: their immunodiagnostic value in Wegener's granulomatosis. Ann Int Med 111:28
43. Schmitt WH, Heesen C, Rautmann A, Gross WL (1991) Elevated serum levels of soluble interleukin-2 receptor in Wegener's granulomatosis: evidence of T-cell activation. Arthritis Rheum 34 (Suppl 9):S71
44. Scully RE, Mark EJ, McNeely WF, McNeely BU (1987) Periarteritis nodosa. N Engl J Med 316:1139–1147
45. Scully RE, Mark EJ, McNeely WF, McNeely BU (1991) Allergic fungal sinusitis. N Engl J Med 324:1423–1429
46. Specks U, DeRemee RA (1990) Granulomatous vasculitis. Rheum Dis Clin North Am 16:377–397
47. Steppat D, Gross WL (1989) Stage-adapted treatment of Wegener's granulomatosis. Klin Wochenschr 67:666–671
48. Travis WD, Kalafer ME, Robin HS, Luibel FJ (1990) Hypersensitivity pneumonitis and pulmonary vasculitis with eosinophilia in a patient taking an L-tryptophan preparation. Ann Intern Med 112:301–302
49. Wegener F (1939) Über eine eigenartige rhinogene Granulomatose mit besonderer Beteiligung des Arteriensystems und der Nieren. Z Pathol Anat 109:36
50. Wegener F (1990) Wegener's granulomatosis: thoughts and observations of a pathologist. Eur Arch Otorhinolaryngol 247:133–142
51. Weidhase A, Grvne HJ, Unterberg C, Schuff-Werner P, Wiegand V (1990) Severe granulomatous giant cell myocarditis in Wegener's granulomatosis. Klin Wochenschr 68:880–885

Isolated Angiitis of the Central Nervous System

Patricia M. Moore

1 Definition

Isolated angiitis of the CNS (IAC) is an idiopathic, recurrent vasculitis restricted to small and medium-sized vessels of the brain and spinal cord. Early reports were based on autopsy cases, but the disease is now increasingly recognized and treated ante mortem. Initially the disease was called "granulomatous angiitis" [2, 5, 6, 8, 10, 11] but the term "isolated angiitis" is preferable because it emphasizes the location of the vasculitis rather than a variable histologic finding. The true incidence is unknown, but the disease is not as rare as previously thought.

2 Pathology

Tissue ischemia is the common denominator of the vasculitides. Both the acutely inflamed and the chronically scarred vessels have narrowed lumens and reduced delivery of blood. Other features of the mononuclear cell inflammation that increase the likelihood of ischemia are the increased procoagulant effects of interleukin-stimulated endothelial cells and potential spasm of the vascular muscularis. In the smaller vessels hemorrhage is more frequently encountered [3]. Factors other than ischemia may contribute to tissue injury. A role for cytokine effects on the parenchyma and edema has been suggested but there is no current evidence for or against either [13, 14].

Pathologically, the disease occurs in small and medium-sized vessels in the CNS within the dural reflections. In the brain the changes are scattered but diffuse, multiple vessels are invariable affected. It is more difficult to determine the extent of involvement of the spinal cord and roots [4]. Likewise, the frequency of changes within the eye remains unexplored; but both choroidal and retinal vasculitis may occur. The infiltrate is usually mononuclear with a variable amount of accompanying polymorphonuclear cells. Immunoglobulin is usually not present in the vessel wall. The extent of necrosis varies, and it is more often described in autopsy than in biopsy series; this may reflect the temporal evolution of the infiltrate or be part of the end stage, chronically scarred arteries late in the course of the disease.

P. Berlit, P. M. Moore (Eds.)
Vasculitis, Rheumatic Disease
and the Nervous System
© Springer-Verlag Berlin Heidelberg 1993

Table 1. Clinical features in IAC

	Frequency (%)
Headaches	75
Encephalopathy	75
Strokes	60–70
Cranial neuropathy	20
Subarachnoid hemorrhage	< 10
Myelopathy	15
Radiculopathy	< 5

3 Clinic

Clinically, the manifestations are protean. Because the small blood vessels may be extensively involved, headaches and encephalopathy are as frequent a presenting manifestation as stroke. Table 1 shows the frequency of clinical findings. The course may be indolent or fulminant but is characteristically recurrent and, untreated, progressive to death within 1–5 years. Headaches may be generalized or localized but are notably severe and throbbing. As the disease progresses, focal deficits typically occur. Multiple localized lesions of the cerebrum, cerebellum, or brainstem are present in more than 75% of patients. Myelopathies, cranial neuropathies, and chronic meningitis are also seen.

Systemic symptoms and signs are notably absent. There is no clinical or laboratory evidence of systemic inflammation. Patients do not have arthralgias, rashes, abdominal pain, or altered renal or hepatic function. If an elevated erythrocyte sedimentation rate, antinuclear antibodies, rheumatoid factor, or immune complexes are present in significant titers, an alternate diagnosis such as chronic infection or systemic collagen vascular disease should be considered. In fact, there are no blood studies to suggest or confirm IAC.

Similarly, the noninvasive neurodiagnostic studies may be abnormal but more often reflect the results of ischemia and stroke rather than the underlying vascular inflammation. Electroencephalograms may display areas of focal slowing or irritability. Computed tomography (CT) scans show parenchymal areas of stroke. Magnetic resonance imaging (MRI) scans may show more (and smaller) areas of stroke but do not reveal the areas of vascular inflammation unassociated with tissue infarction. Even MRI angiography does not currently have the resolution to show the multifocal, scattered, vascular changes.

4 Diagnosis

A diagnosis of isolated angiitis of the CNS depends on angiography and biopsy. Cerebral angiography is the earliest and sometimes the only abnormal neurodiagnostic study. Typical angiographic abnormalities include mul-

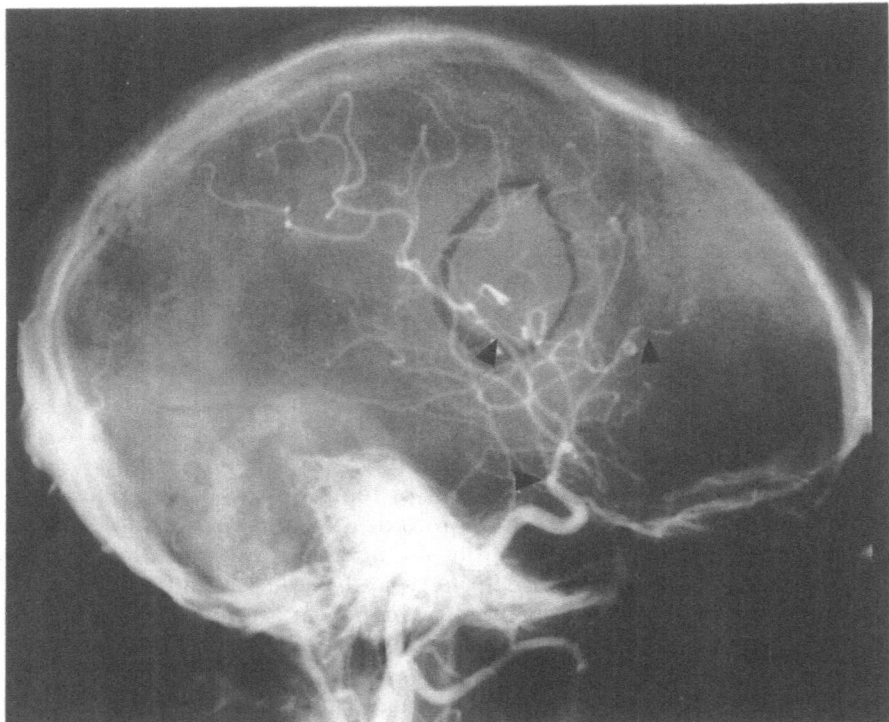

Fig. 1. Carotid angiography showing several areas of segmental narrowing, indicated by the arrowheads

tiple localized areas of narrowing, occlusion of vessels, delayed emptying of vessels, and anastomotic channels (Fig. 1). There is no predilection for bifurcations and aneurysms are atypical, in contrast to systemic vasculitis. Angiograms are not invariably abnormal. Patients with histologic evidence of vasculitis may have normal angiograms, even with magnification studies, when the disease is confined to small vessels beyond the resolution of angiography. Nor are any angiographic features pathognomonic for IAC. The larger group of secondary vasculitides and a wide range of vasculopathies may initially appear similar to IAC.

Tissue biopsy is the most specific diagnostic test for vasculitis. A wedge parenchymal and leptomeningeal sample is usually removed from the non-dominant hemisphere (Fig. 2). Biopsy is needed not only to confirm the presence of inflammation but to exclude alternate diagnoses such as infections, neoplasia, amyloidosis, and other causes of vasculopathy. The procedure has been safe and effective with the strongest limitation of a false negative result that appears to be more frequent, as anticipated, early in the course of the disease.

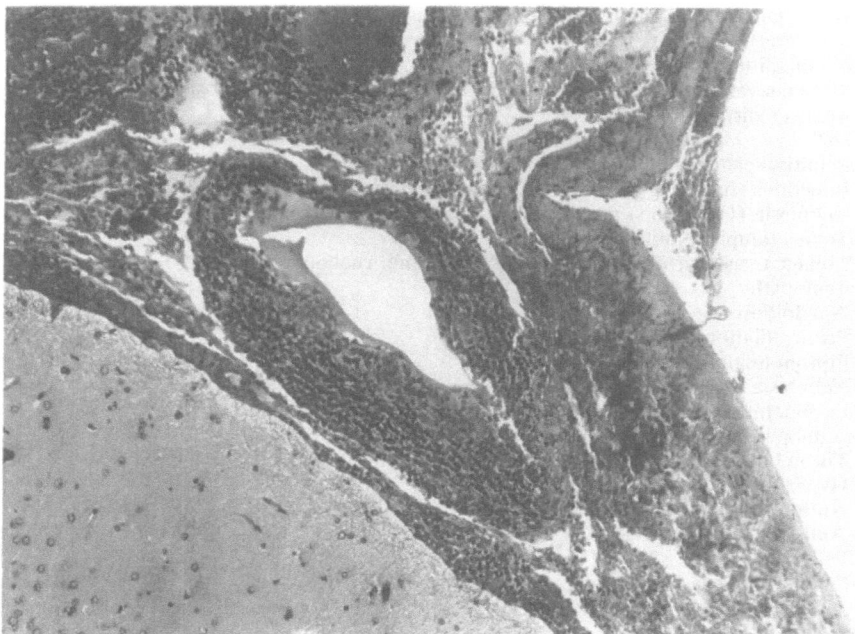

Fig. 2. Leptomeningeal/parenchymal biopsy showing dense infiltrate in small artery

5 Differential Diagnosis

Differential diagnosis of IAC includes the much larger group of primary and secondary vasculopathies (Table 2). In this group, systemic idiopathic and secondary vasculitides are important because the CNS may be the presenting manifestation of disease. Diagnosis depends on carefully delineating the extent of even preclinical vascular changes (by creatine clearance and retinal angiography for example). Because infections are an important cause of vasculitis [7, 9, 12, 16, 19], fungi, in particular, need to be excluded by culture of tissue.

Other vascular diseases are not inflammatory. Amyloid, postirradiation changes, and lymphoma are examples of processes which may affect blood vessels and cause focal CNS lesions, usually with angiographic abnormalities, but are distinct entities, different from IAC [5, 18]. Other disorders affect coagulation so the vessels themselves are only secondarily involved in thrombosis. In this group are included hyperviscosity syndromes, sickle cell disease, anti-factor VIII-associated strokes [1], and some anticardiolipin-associated strokes.

6 Pathogenesis and Etiology

The cause of isolated angiitis remains unknown. The presence of a predominantly mononuclear cell infiltrate and occasional granulomas, and the

Table 2. Differential diagnosis of CNS vasculitis

Vasculitis, idiopathic
   Systemic vasculitis (polyarteritis nodosa, Wegener's granulomatosis)
   Behçet's disease
   IAC
Vasculitis, secondary
   Infections (fungi, viral, bacterial, treponemal, mycobacterial)
   Neoplasia (Hodgkin's, paraneoplasic)
   Toxins (amphetamines, cocaine)
   Collagen vascular disease (Sjögren's syndrome, rheumatoid arthritis)
Vasculopathy
   Amyloidosis
   Postirradiation
   Fibromuscular dysplasia
   Neoplasia (lymphoma)
   Degenerative (systemic lupus erythematosus)
Coagulopathy
   Thrombocytic thrombocytopenic purpura
   Hyperviscosity
   Antiphospholipid/cardiolipin antibody
   Anti-factor VII antibody
   Paraproteinemia
   Sickle cell disease

---

absence of antibodies or immune complexes in the vessel wall, suggest a disorder of cell-mediated immunity [17]. The reason for the activation of the cell-mediated immune system is not clear. There are no clinical, serologic, or hereditary features characteristic of an underlying collagen vascular disease. The occurrence of a histologically similar vasculitis in some patients with Hodgkin's disease [5] or herpes zoster [12] has suggested an underlying neoplastic or viral pathogenesis. To date, no patient with IAC has had clinical or serologic evidence of a viral infection, immunosuppression does not activate a latent virus, nor has an infection become manifest in more than 10 years of follow-up of some patients. Similarly, neoplasia has not developed in patients with IAC followed over time.

The absence of histologic differences in the vessels of patients with inflammatory diseases of diverse etiology does not exclude the presence of distinct subsets. Current information shows that we can maximize our information about underlying processes by a careful history and physical exam with focus on the eyes, skin, kidneys and other visceral organs. Historical details should be addressed perupiously about possible toxins including street drugs as well as over the counter and prescribed medications. Laboratory studies should be directed at detecting underlying systemic inflammation or a collagen vascular disease. Biopsy is needed to demonstrate inflammation and, more important, to exclude alternate diseases including infection and neoplasia.

7 Diagnostic Criteria

The current criteria used to establish an ante mortem diagnosis of IAC are:
1. Clinical picture of headaches and multifocal neurologic deficits present for at least 6 months unless the onset is devastating or rapidly progressive
2. Cerebral angiography demonstrating several areas of arterial narrowing
3. Exclusion of systemic infection or inflammation
4. Leptomeningeal/parenchymal biopsy to demonstrate vascular inflammation and to exclude infection, neoplasia, and primary vasculopathies.

We recognize an occasional patient with normal angiogram or non diagnostic biopsy.

8 Treatment

IAC is treated with a combination of cyclophosphamide and low- to medium-dose corticosteroids (maintenance equivalence 20 mg prednisone/day). Corticosteroids alone have been ineffective in acute stages of disease and are associated with a high rate of relapse in quiescent disease [11]. High dosages of corticosteroids have numerous side effects, including an angiotoxic potential. Other regimens of immunosuppression including methotrexate have not resulted in remissions of symptoms. Cyclophosphamide is effective in both acute events and in prevention of recurrence. Both oral and the intravenous bolus routes are effective. Treatment must include rigorous attention to both the white blood cell count and the presence of blood in the urine. The goal of therapy is to prevent recurrent ischemic attacks; headaches are frequently a useful, but not infallible guide to disease activity. Leukopenia, particularly neutropenia, is the limitation not the goal of therapy. The dosage is titered to the clinical effects but a minimum of 1 year's therapy appears to prevent recurrence. Repeat angiography is useful to determine whether the lesions are stable, improving, or increasing in number. We continue therapy until the patient is clinically asymptomatic for 1 year and the angiographic lesions have stabilized or resolved.

The diagnosis and treatment of CNS vasculitis requires the skills of a general clinician and the knowledge of a specialist. Our approach to patients with possible CNS vasculitis will continue to evolve as we better understand the pathogenic mechanisms and devise more specific and less toxic therapies.

References

1. Belch JJF, Zoma AA, Richards IM, Mclaughlin K, Forbes CD, Sturrock RD (1987) Vascular damage and factor-VIII-related antigen in the rheumatic diseases. Rheumatol Int 7:107–111
2. Burger PC, Burch JG, Vogel FS (1977) Granulomatous angiitis. An unusual etiology of stroke. Stroke 8:29–35

3. Edwards KR (1977) Hemorrhagic complications of cerebral arteritis. Arch Neurol 34:549–552
4. Feasby TE, Ferguson GG, Kaufman JCE (1975) Isolated spinal cord arteritis. Can J Neurol Sci 2:143–146
5. Greco FA, Kolins J, Rajjoub RK, Brereton HD (1976) Hodgkin's disease and granulomatous angiitis of the central nervous system. Cancer 38:2027–2032
6. Hughes JT, Brownell B (1966) Granulomatous giant-celled angiitis of the central nervous system. Neurology 16:293–298
7. Igarashi M, Gilmartin RC, Gerald B, Wilburn F, Jabbour JT (1984) Cerebral arteritis and bacterial meningitis. Arch Neurol 41:531–535
8. Jellinger K (1977) Giant cell granulomatous angiitis of the central nervous system. J Neurol 215:175–190
9. Koeppen AH, Lansing LS, Peng S, Smith RS (1981) Central nervous system vasculitis in cytomegalovirus infection. J Neurosci 51:395–410
10. Kolodny EH, Rebeiz JJ, Caviness VS Jr, Richardson EP Jr (1968) Granulomatous angiitis of the central nervous system. Arch Neurol 19:510–524
11. Koo EH, Massey EW (1988) Granulomatous angiitis of the central nervous system: protean manifestations and response to treatment. J Neurol Neurosurg Psychiatry 51:1126–1133
12. Linnemann CC, Alvira MM (1980) Pathogenesis of varicella-zoster angiitis in the CNS. Arch Neurol 37:239–240
13. Male D, Pryce G, Hughes C, Lantos P (1990) Lymphocyte migration into brain modelled in vitro: control by lymphocyte actication, cytokines, and antigen. Cell Immunol 127:1–11
14. Mannik M (1987) Experimental models for immune complex-mediated vascular inflammation. Acad Med Scand Suppl 715:145–155
15. Moore PM (1989) Diagnosis and management of isolated angiitis of the central nervous system. Neurology 39:167–173
16. Moore PM, Cupps TR (1983) Neurological complications of vasculitis. Ann Neurol 14:155–167
17. Moore PM (1989) Immune mechanisms in the primary and secondary vasculitides. J Neurol Sci 93:129–145
18. Rager-Zisman B (1988) Virus-induced autoimmunity. First Auto Meet-Sto Day 244 no 7:363–365
19. Ramos M, Mandybur TI (1975) Cerebral vasculitis in rheumatoid arthritis. Arch Neurol 32:271–275
20 Roeitgen DP, Weimer GR, Patterson LF (1981) Delayed neurologic complications of left atrial myxoma. Neurology 31:8–13
21. Sergent JS, Christian CL (1974) Necrotizing vasculitis after acute serous otitis media. Ann Int Med 81:195–199

Neuropsychiatric Disorders in Systemic Lupus Erythematosus

Harry G. Bluestein

1 The Clinical Spectrum of SLE

"Lupus can do everything ..." is the beginning of an aphorism emphasizing the broad spectrum of clinical manifestations that may occur in patients with systemic lupus erythematosus (SLE). Neuropsychiatric abnormalities are frequent, occurring in 40%–50% of all patients with lupus at some time during the course of their illness [2, 11, 13].

Nervous system involvement is like a microcosm of the systemic illness in that it, too, can present with a wide variety of manifestations. Virtually any sign or symptom of neuropathology can be seen in SLE, ranging from defects in the highest cerebral functions of reasoning, memory, and reality testing, through gross disturbances of cortical motor function, abnormal motor regulation by the cerebellum and basal ganglia, involvement of the spinal cord, cranial and peripheral neuropathies, to abnormalities at the neuromuscular junction [4].

Diffuse CNS involvement in the form of encephalopathies, with or without psychosis, and generalized seizures are the most prototypic manifestations. The presentations are usually dramatic or even awesome in patients with florid psychosis. Yet this striking clinical picture may improve rapidly in response to therapy or as part of the natural course of the illness and leave no sign of residual nervous system damage.

Focal lesions in the nervous system in the form of cranial or peripheral neuropathies, cerebrovascular accidents, chorea, and transverse myelitis also occur, and many patients with nervous system involvement exhibit more than one manifestation. Half of them will have psychiatric as well as neurologic problems. Thus, nervous system involvement is due to pathogenic mechanisms that can cause multifocal impairment of neurologic function at anatomically distinct sites as well as readily reversible diffuse impairment of higher cerebral function.

2 Pathogenesis of Neuro-SLE

Immunopathologic studies in animal models of SLE as well as human tissues have documented the importance of immune complex-mediated vasculitis in

P. Berlit, P. M. Moore (Eds.)
Vasculitis, Rheumatic Disease
and the Nervous System
© Springer-Verlag Berlin Heidelberg 1993

producing multi-organ system damage in SLE. Neuropsychiatric problems had been attributed to similar mechanisms, thus accounting for the clinical use of the terms "CNS vasculitis" and "lupus cerebritis" as shorthand names for those manifestations. However, true vasculitis, with inflammatory cells invading vessel walls and fibrinoid necrosis, so characteristic of the small artery involvement found in the kidney and other tissues of SLE, is infrequent in autopsy studies of the brain [10, 15].

Although vasculitis is unusual, central nervous tissue from patients who succumbed to the neuropsychiatric effects of SLE commonly show signs of vasculopathy. These include noninflammatory vascular changes, including the vascular endothelial cell membranes. By whatever mechanism the damage occurs, the anatomic location of the bland vasculopathy often differs from the neurologic site responsible for the clinical findings. Thus, the changes in the vascular supply to the nervous system are not sufficient by themselves to account for most of the neuropsychiatric manifestations of SLE.

In recent years, the search for additional pathogenic mechanisms participating in the development of CNS lupus has focused on the importance of autoantibodies reactive with neuronal membrane antigens. There are precedents in SLE for a pathogenic role for membrane-reactive autoantibodies. Antibodies to blood elements contribute to hemolytic anemia, thrombocytopenia, and lymphopenia. Interestingly, autoimmune hematologic problems occur more frequently in patients with neuropsychiatric involvement than in other lupus patients. Neuron-reactive antibodies are also frequently detected in SLE sera, and there is some evidence that the titers of those antibodies vary with lupus activity in the nervous system [1, 2, 7, 8, 14, 25]. An autoantibody-mediated pathogenesis is an attractive explanation for the diffuse and reversible manifestations of the more common neuropsychiatric features of SLE.

3 Pathogenic Role of Neuron-Reactive Antibodies

The potential pathogenic role of neuron-reactive antibodies is supported by the observation that these antibodies are present within the nervous system of lupus patients with CNS disease. In fact, neuron-reactive antibodies of the immunoglobulin G class are present in cerebrospinal fluid (CSF) of patients with active neuropsychiatric involvement and not other lupus patients [5, 26]. The association is particularly strong in those patients with encephalopathies, psychosis, and seizures. The measurement of immunoglobulin G neuron-reactive antibodies in CSF is also a valuable diagnostic test. It is sensitive, elevated in 75% of all lupus patients with CNS involvement (neuro-SLE) and in more than 90% of those with diffuse involvement (encephalopathy with or without psychosis and seizures); and it is specific, negative in 95% of lupus patients without clinically apparent neuropsychiatric involvement.

The immunoglobulin G neuron-reactive antibodies do not appear to be exerting their effects via a cytotoxic mechanism. Cell death is not seen on pathologic examinations. Thus, the most common diffuse neuropsychiatric manifestations of SLE appear to result from the binding of autoantibodies to molecules on neuronal membranes, thereby interfering with the cells' ability to respond to or propagate neural signals. The neuron-reactive antibodies probably enter the CNS through an impaired blood–brain barrier – most likely via immunologically damaged cerebral vessels – but in some cases may be produced locally within the nervous system.

The pathogenic significance of membrane-reactive antibodies that may affect the function of the nervous system has led to a search for the target molecules of those antibodies with the expectation that their identification will provide clues to the mechanisms for functional disruption. The best-defined neuronal molecules that are targets of SLE antibodies are the ribosomal P proteins [6, 9, 22] and neurofilaments [19, 20]. Elevated levels of immunoglobulin G antibodies to those molecules correlate with the diffuse CNS lupus manifestations. Antiribosomal P protein antibodies are relatively specific for severe psychiatric disturbances (psychosis or profound depression), while the antineurofilament antibodies are associated with encephalopathies and generalized seizures as well as psychoses.

A direct effect of lupus neuron-reactive antibodies on neuronal function has not yet been documented. Experiments in animals, however, have documented that antibodies to CNS antigens can induce pathologic changes in the nervous system and alterations in behavior that are quite similar to those that characterize lupus CNS involvement. When injected into spinal fluid of normal rabbits, antibodies to brain produce foci of cerebral edema accompanied by motor discoordination and epileptic seizures [23]. Similarly, antibody to synaptosomal plasma membranes caused significant memory impairment, while intracerebral injection of antibodies to brain gangliosides generated seizures in rats [17, 18]. Thus there is a reasonable basis for implicating antibodies reactive with molecules on neuronal membranes in the pathogenesis of neuropsychiatric dysfunction.

A pathogenic role for antibodies directed at intracytoplasmic molecules in neurons is less plausible. In vivo, the intact membrane of the living cells prevents interaction between the antibody and its target intracellular antigen, unless, of course, the antigen itself or another molecule expressing cross-reactive epitopes is also present on the cell surface. In the case of ribosomal P proteins and neurofilaments, there is some evidence that antibodies to those molecules react with neuronal cell membranes. In a preliminary study, affinity-purified antibody to ribosomal P protein bound specifically to the surface of live cultured neuroblastoma cells [16]. Similarly, a monoclonal antibody to the high molecular weight neurofilament protein isolated from the serum of a patient with an immunoglobulin A monoclonal gammopathy cross-reacts with 65 kDa protein expressed on the membrane of neuroblastoma cells [21]. The membrane-bound molecules reactive with the antiribosomal P and antineurofilament antibodies have not yet been fully characterized, but preliminary evidence suggests that they are not identical to, but share epitopes with, the intracytoplasmic molecules.

4 Diagnostic Value of Neuron-Reactive Antibodies

Independent of their role in the pathogenesis of CNS lupus, the neuron-reactive antibodies play an important role in diagnosis. The assay of membrane-reactive immunoglobulin G antineuronal antibody in the spinal fluid is the most sensitive and specific test for the diagnosis of the diffuse neuropsychiatric manifestations of neuro-SLE [5, 26]. Antibodies to ribosomal P proteins have a narrower specificity for severe psychiatric disturbances. In a comparison of those two tests in a small number of patients, the antiribosomal P assay was less sensitive than the antineuronal membrane assay even in those patients with psychosis [24]. There were no patients in that study with severe depression where the antiribosomal P assay is very sensitive [22], but the antineuronal binding assay in CSF has generally not been abnormal in patients whose only neuropsychiatric manifestation is depression. Thus, the antiribosomal P protein assay may be most useful for implicating lupus as the cause of that psychiatric problem.

These antineuronal antibody assays are becoming more widely available in commercial laboratories. Their appropriate role in the diagnosis of neuropsychiatric lupus will evolve as experience with them increases.

5 Conclusions

SLE is considered the nec plus ultra of autoimmune diseases because of the broad spectrum of organ pathology it can produce. To a large degree, the multisystemic involvement can be attributed to the immune complex vasculitis in the affected organs. However, that immunopathologic process is generally not a feature of nervous system involvement, particularly in its most common aspects, encephalopathies, psychoses and seizures. A strong association of antineuronal antibodies with the clinically apparent neuropsychiatric manifestations of SLE; the occasionally documented rise in antineuronal activity just prior to the onset of lupus CNS disease; and the absence of those antibodies in similar kinds of neuropsychiatric dysfunction associated with other disorders provides strong circumstantial evidence in support of the hypothesis that neuron-reactive antibodies participate in the pathogenesis of neuropsychiatric dysfunction. Identification of the specific membrane molecules that are the target of the pathogenic antibodies and the mechanisms by which antibody interaction with those molecules deters neurologic function will be needed for the development of more effective strategies for the treatment and prevention of these problems.

References

1. Avinoach I, Amitel-Teplizki H, Kuperman O, Isenberg DA, Shoenfeld Y (1990) Characteristics of antineuronal antibodies in systemic lupus erythematosus patients with and without central nervous system involvement: the role of mycobacterial cross-reacting antigens. Israel J Med Sci 26:367–373
2. Baker M (1973) Psychopathology in SLE. Semin Arthritis Rheum 3:95
3. Bluestein HG (1978) Neurocytotoxic antibodies in serum of patients with systemic lupus erythematosus. Proc Natl Acad Sci USA 75:396
4. Bluestein HG (1991) Neuropsychiatric disorders in systemic lupus erythematosus. In: Lahita RG (ed) Systemic lupus erythematosus. Wiley, Chichester
5. Bluestein HG, Williams GW, Steinberg AD (1981) Cerebrospinal fluid antibodies to neuronal cells. Association with neuropsychiatric manifestations of systemic lupus erythematosus. Am J Med 70:240
6. Bonfa E, Golombek SJ, Kaufmann LD et al (1987) Association between lupus erythematosus and anti-ribosomal P protein antibodies. N Engl J Med 317:265
7. Bresnihan B, Oliver M, Williams B et al. (1979) An antineuronal antibody cross-reactive with erythrocytes and lymphocytes in systemic lupus erythematosus. Arthritis Rheum 22:313
8. Danon YL, Garty BZ (1986) Autoantibodies to neuroblastoma cell surface antigens in neuropsychiatric lupus. Neuropediatrics 17:23–27
9. Elkon KB, Skelly S, Parnassa AP, Moller W, Danko W, Weissbach H, Brot N (1986) Identification and chemical synthesis of a ribosomal protein antigenic determinant in systemic lupus erythematosus. Proc Natl Acad Sci USA 83:7419–7423
10. Ellis SG, Verity MA (1979) Central nervous system involvement in sytemic lupus erythematosus: a review of neuropathologic findings in 57 cases (1955–1977). Semin Arthritis Rheum 8:212
11. Estes D, Christian CL (1971) The natural history of SLE by prospective analysis. Medicine 50:85
12. Fabian RH (1990) Uptake of antineuronal IgM by CNS neurons: comparison with antineuronal IgG. Neurology 40:419–422
13. Harvey AM, Shulman LE, Tumulty A, et al. (1954) Systemic lupus erythematosus: review of the literature and clinical analysis of 138 cases. Medicine 33:291
14. How A, Dent PD, Liao SK, Denburg JD (1985) Antineuronal antibodies in neuropsychiatric systemic lupus erythematosus. Arthritis Rheum 28:789–795
15. Johnson RT, Richardson EP (1968) The neurologic manifestations of systemic lupus erythematosus: a clinical-pathological study of 24 cases and review of the literature. Medicine 47:337
16. Karen E, Reichlin MW, Koscec M, Fugate RD, Reichlin M (1991) Autoantibodies to the ribrosomal P protein react with a plasma membrane related target on human cells. Arthritis Rheum 34:S75
17. Karpiak SE, Graf L, Rappaport MM (1976) Antiserum to brain gangliosides produces recurrent epileptiform activity. Science 194:735
18. Kobiler D, Fuchs S, Samuel D (1976) The effect of antisynaptosomal plasma membrane antibodies on memory. Brain Res 115:129
19. Kurki P, Helve T, Dahl D, Virtanen I (1986) Neurofilament antibodies in systemic lupus erythematosus. Rheumatology 13:69–73
20. Robbins ML, Korngut SE, Bell CL, Kalinke T, England D, Turski P, Graziano FM (1988) Antineurofilament antibody evaluation in neuropsychiatric SLE. Combination with anticardiolipin antibody assay and MRI. Arthritis Rheum 31:623–631
21. Sadiq SA, van den Berg LH, Kilidereas K, Harp AP, Latov N (1991) Human monoclonal antineurofilament antibody cross-reacts with an neuronal surface protein. J Neurosci Res 29:319–325
22. Schneebaum AB, Singleton JD, West SG, Blodgett JK, Allen LG, Cheronis JC, Kotzin BL (1991) Association of psychiatric manifestations with antibodies to ribrosomal P proteins in systemic in lupus erythematosus. Am J Med 90:54–62

23. Simon J, Simon O (1975) Effect of passive transfer of anti-brain antibodies to a normal recipient. Exp Neurol 47:523
24. Spezialetti R, Peter JB, Bluestein HG (1990) Clinical correlations between anti-ribosomal P and anti-neuronal cell antibodies in CNS-SLE. Arthritis Rheum 33:S102
25. Wilson HA, Winfield JB, Lahita RG et al. (1979) Association of IgG antibrain antibodies with central nervous system dysfunction in systemic lupus erythematosus. Arthritis Rheum 22:458
26. Zhang N-Z, Chen WZ (1989) Antineuronal antibodies in Chinese patients with neuropsychiatric SLE. Proceedings of the second international conference on systemic lupus erythematosus. Professional Postgraduate Services, Tokyo, p 109

Psychiatric Syndromes Associated with Vasculitis

Karl-Ludwig Täschner

1 Psychopathologic Syndromes in Neurologic Disease

The occurrence of psychopathologic syndromes in patients with physical pathology is not rare. We are indebted to Bonhoeffer for having classified the psychoses into two basic categories early in this century [4, 15]. The first category includes psychoses without any detectable physical cause, while the second includes those due to exogenous factors. Bonhoeffer designated the latter the "exogenous reactive" type, the term still used today.

Originally it was assumed that the symptomatology of the psychoses would be uniform, in view of the widely differing effects on the CNS. However, we now know that there are many syndromes which cannot be ascribed exclusively to individual physical disorders. Thus, when considering the exogenous psychoses we are confronted with a caleidoscope of psychopathologic symptoms, and the lack of uniformity in the nomenclature can only serve to increase the confusion. Today, we know that there is no such thing as "the organic psychosis," because the symptoms can vary very widely and almost all known individual psychiatric syndromes can also occur in organic psychoses.

On this subject Weitbrecht [28], in his treatise "Zur Frage der Spezifität psychopathologischer Symptome" (On the question of the specificity of psychopathologic symptoms, 1957) wrote the following: "We cannot name a single psychopathologic symptom which is specific to a particular psychosis such that its presence would permit a disease entity to be diagnosed with certainty."

Referring to Fleck [9], he goes on to explain that even clouding of consciousness is not necessarily a symptom of the exogenous reactive form. In the past 20 years this view has been fully confirmed through the investigation of the great complex of drug-induced psychoses [25, 26]. This, incidentally, has given rise to numerous hypotheses concerning the origins of the endogenous psychoses.

However, this also highlights a problem which has been given comparatively little attention in psychiatry. If all symptoms are nonspecific the distinction between different disease entities is also unclear. Therefore, specific psychoses cannot be expected to be associated with a specific underlying organic pathology.

P. Berlit, P. M. Moore (Eds.)
Vasculitis, Rheumatic Disease
and the Nervous System
© Springer-Verlag Berlin Heidelberg 1993

2 Psychiatric Symptoms and Vasculitis

As early as 1872, Kaposi [16] pointed out that lupus erythematosus can be associated with mental changes, but little attention was paid to the problem until a century later. In 1972, in the second edition of the manual "Psychiatrie der Gegenwart," Conrad [8] wrote: "There is increasing evidence that some psychoses originate from rheumatic angiitis of the brain, and that their course can correspond exactly to that of a schizophrenic process." He referred in this context to the work of Bruetsch [6], who had studied these psychoses particularly in connection with thromboangiitis obliterans.

Since then there have been several publications on the subject. The study by Meyer [21] on the psychopathology of thromboangiitis deserves a brief mention. He distinguished three groups of patients. The first, with mainly neurologic symptoms, are of no interest in the present context. The second group comprises cases with cerebral atrophy. In some of these patients an exaggeration of the personality was observed, in others a deterioration of the personality to the point of dementia. Cognitive disorders, slowness of movement, decreased energy, moodiness, and delirious images may also be part of the picture. Meyer [21] also claimed that "schizophrenic symptomatology" was by no means uncommon, and that disturbances of consciousness also occurred. Finally, Meyer's third group comprises patients with a combination of neurologic and psychiatric changes, who he claims can be distinguished by a peculiar segmentation pattern of both the capillaries and larger vessels. Huber [14] also discusses Meyer's study in his contribution to the manual.

3 Psychosis and Lupus Erythematosus

The classification of the various psychopathologic syndromes in systemic lupus erythematosus (SLE) differs from author to author and from sample to sample. In most cases cerebro-organic syndromes in encephalopathy dominate, followed by schizophreniform psychoses and depressions [22–24]. Other authors put the depressions in second [17] or even in first place [12]. Estimates of the percentage of SLE cases involving psychoses differ widely. Guze [12] gave a figure of 24%, while Ganz [11] put it at 56%. Estimates as low as 3% and as high as 65% have also been made [1, 10, 20, 27] (see Table 1).

The premorbid personality structure clearly plays a major role in the occurrence of psychosis in SLE, but external stress factors are also of importance. This brings us to the vulnerability model proposed by Häfner [13]. Naturally, steroid therapy should also be born in mind, since glucocorticoids have long been thought to produce psychoses. However, it is usually prescribed in high doses only for relatively serious conditions. The question of a causal relationship in these circumstances is therefore always somewhat problematic [20].

Table 1. Distribution of psychiatric disorders in SLE patients
(as percentages of the total number of female SLE patients with psychiatric disorders)

	Krüger (1984) [17]	Nakano and Miyashima (1983) [22]	Guze (1967) [12]	Ganz et al. (1972) [11]
Organic syndromes (exogenic reaction types)	25	44	9	22
Affective syndromes (esp. depressive symptoms)	22	20	10	
Schizophreniform syndromes	5	28	5	35
Mixed syndromes	15			

Recent studies in the Far East [18, 22] have also drawn attention to the problem of psychiatric disease in SLE. Encephalopathies and schizophreniform psychoses also predominate there; depressions are less common. A case of catatonia has also been described [19], and Berlit and coworkers [2, 3] have likewise published studies on the subject. Their suggestion that lithium, antipsychotics, and anticonvulsants can cause drug-induced SLE should at least be considered, if not investigated, in psychiatric patients with some of the features of SLE. This comes close to suggesting reciprocity – SLE caused by psychotropic drugs, psychotropic drugs to treat psychoses, psychoses following SLE. When we also learn that psychiatric symptoms can precede the manifestation of SLE by up to 10 years [7], the prospects with regard to the possible side effects of antipsychotics hardly bear thinking about. In these cases in particular, the value of the determination of neuronreactive autoantibodies, which have a great sensitivity in the detection of diffuse CNS involvement in SLE, becomes evident [5].

References

1. Andrew WF (1975) Psychiatric illness associated with systemic lupus erythematodes. Am Med J 68:1207–1210
2. Berlit P (1989) Lupus erythematodes und Nervensystem. Dtsch Ärztebl 86:3176–3182
3. Berlit P, Kessler CH, Storch B, Krause KH (1983) Immunvaskulitis und Nervensystem. Nervenarzt 54:497–503
4. Bleuler M. Willi J, Bühler HR (1966) Akute psychische Begleiterscheinungen körperlicher Krankheiten. Akuter exogener Reaktionstypus. Übersicht und neue Forschungen. Thieme, Stuttgart
5. Bluestein HG, Williams GW, Steinberg AD (1981) Cerebrospinal fluid antibodies to neuronal cells: association with neuropsychiatric manifestations of systemic lupus erythematosus. Am J Med 70:240
6. Bruetsch WL (1939) Chronische und rheumatische Gehirnerkrankung als Ursache von Geisteskrankheiten. Eine klinisch-anatomische Studie. Z Neurol 166:4

7. Brun A, Gustafson L (1988) Zerebrovaskuläre Erkrankungen. In: Kisker KP, Lauter H, Meyer JE, Müller C, Strömgren E (eds) Psychiatrie der Gegenwart, vol 6, Organische Psychosen, 3rd edn. Springer, Berlin Heidelberg New York, pp 253–295

8. Conrad K (1972) Die symptomatischen Psychosen. In: Kisker KP, Meyer JE, Müller M, Strömgren E (eds) Psychiatrie der Gegenwart, vol II/2, 2nd edn. Springer, Berlin Heidelberg New York, pp 1–70

9. Fleck U (1956) Über die Bewubtseinstrübung bei den exogenen Reaktionsformen (Bonhoeffer). Nervenarzt 27:433–440

10. Foerster K, Foerster G, Glatzel J (1976) Symptomatische Schizophrenie bei Lupus erythematodes disseminatus. Nervenarzt 47:265–267

11. Ganz VH, Gurland BJ, Deming WE (1972) The study of the psychiatric symptoms of SLE. Psychosom Med 34:207–220

12. Guze SB (1967) The occurence of psychiatric illness in systemic lupus erythematosus. Am J Psychiatry 123:1562–1570

13. Häfner H (1989) Ist Schizophrenie eine Krankheit? Nervenarzt 60:191–199

14. Huber G (1972) Klinik und Psychopathologie der organischen Psychosen. In: Kisker KP, Meyer JE, Müller M. Strömgren E (eds) Psychiatrie der Gegenwart, vol II/2, 2nd edn. Springer, Berlin Heidelberg New York, pp 71–146

15. Huber G (1988) Körperlich begründbare psychische Störungen bei Intoxikationen, Allgemein- und Stoffwechselstörungen, bei inneren und dermatologischen Erkrankungen, Endokrinopathien, Generationsvorgängen, Vitaminmangel und Hirntumoren. In: Kisker KP, Lauter H, Meyer JE, Müller C, Strömgren E (eds) Psychiatrie der Gegenwart, vol 6, Organische Psychosen, 3rd edn. Springer, Berlin Heidelberg New York, pp 198–252

16. Kaposi MK (1872) New findings in lupus erythematosus. Arch Dermatol Syph 4:36

17. Krüger KW (1984) Lupus erythematodes und Zentralnervensystem. Nervenarzt 55:165–172

18. Lim LC, Lee TE, Boey ML (1991) Psychiatric manifestations of systemic lupus erythematosus in Singapore – a cross-cultural comparison. Br J Psychiatry 159:520–523

19. Mac DS, Pardo MP (1983) Systemic lupus erythematosus and catatonia: a case report. J Clin Psychiatry 44:155–156

20. McNeill A, Grennan DM, Ward D, Dick WC (1976) Psychiatric problems in systemic lupus erythematosus. Br J Psychiatry 128:442–445

21. Meyer HH (1953) Die cerebrale Thrombangiitis obliterans. Fortschr Neurol Psychiatr 21:201–222

22. Nakano T, Miyasaka M (1983) On the recent trend of psychiatric symptoms in systemic lupus erythematosus – from experiences after 1975. Psychiatr Neurol Jpn 85:348

23. O'Connor JF (1959) Psychoses associated with disseminated lupus erythematosus. Ann Intern Med 51:526–536

24. Stern M, Robbins ES (1960) Psychosis in systemic lupus erythematosus. Arch Gen Psychiatry 3:205–212

25. Täschner KL (1980) Rausch und Psychose – Psychopathologische Untersuchungen an Drogenkonsumenten. Kohlhammer, Stuttgart

26. Täschner KL (1983) Zur Psychopathologie und Differentialdiagnose sogenannter Cannabispsychosen. Fortschr Neurol Psychiatr 51:235–248

27. Waring EM (1972) Psychiatric manifestations of lupus erythematosus. Can Psychiatr Ass J 17:23–27

28. Weitbrecht J (1957) Zur Frage der Spezifität psychopathologischer Symptome. Fortschr Neurol Psychiatr 25:41–56

Treatment of Vasculitides Affecting the Central Nervous System

Patricia M. Moore and *Norbert Gretz*

1 Introduction

Vasculitis is being increasingly recognized as a cause of neurologic disease. The results of treatment vary from excellent to frustrating depending on the type of vasculitis, the etiology, and the stage of the disease. Some regimens in individual diseases dramatically reduce morbidity and mortality. In other disorders the optimal treatment remains empiric.

The general guidelines to therapy are:
1. Treat any precipitating causes such as infections or toxins in the secondary vasculitides.
2. Use the current standard treatment in those primary vasculitides with known responsiveness to specific therapies (prednisone in temporal arteritis and prednisone/cyclophosphamide in Wegener's granulomatosis, polyarteritis nodosa, and isolated angiitis of the CNS)
3. Compare the benefit–risk ratio for treatment in each patient, and begin with the least toxic therapy for the primary vasculitides with responsiveness in less well defined diseases such as lymphomatoid granulomatosus and Behcet's disease.
4. Remember that in the later stages of vasculitic disease, ischemia may result from chronic scarring rather than acute inflammation. This is not responsive to immunosuppressive therapy and the patient should be spared the side effects of ineffective medication.

A brief review of mechanisms of the treatments often used in vasculitis of the nervous system follows. Several other useful reviews are available [4, 5, 8, 22, 25, 29].

2 Prednisone

Glucocorticoids are a cornerstone of therapy in the vasculitic syndromes. Steroids bind to a cytoplasmic receptor protein and enter the cells where they alter the rate of ribosomal and messenger RNA synthesis. This results in modification of the synthesis of specific proteins. Intercellularly, corticosteroids effect numerous important changes in the immune system, including

P. Berlit, P. M. Moore (Eds.)
Vasculitis, Rheumatic Disease
and the Nervous System
© Springer-Verlag Berlin Heidelberg 1993

inhibition of recruitment and migration of neutrophils, lymphocytes, and macrophages to the sites of inflammation and suppression of macrophage chemotaxis, cytotoxicity, and soluble mediator function. They inhibit the production of lymphokines, notably interleukin-2 (IL-2), thereby diminishing the expansion of effector T-cell clones. In vivo, corticosteroids effect both primary and secondary humoral antibody formation in steroid-sensitive species. The primary response is much more sensitive to corticosteroids than the secondary response. Cell-mediated immune reactions are diminished by corticosteroids at several points in the pathway of recruitment of effector cells. The specific effect whereby they ameliorate vasculitic lesions, if indeed there is only one, is uncertain.

The efficacy of glucocorticoids, usually prednisone or methylprednisolone, varies among the vasculitic syndromes. Undoubtedly it is the single most effective treatment in temporal arteritis. In some hypersensitivity vasculitides and in microangiopathic renal vasculitis, prednisone therapy alone may suffice. In other disorders prednisone is used as adjunct therapy, either because it is ineffective as solo therapy or because the high dosage when used as solo therapy is unsustainable due to the considerable side effects. Corticosteroid therapy alone is ineffective in well-established Wegener's granulomatosis. Patients with polyarteritis nodosa may develop new neurologic symptoms while their disease is apparently quiescent on prednisone. It is, however, not yet determined whether all patients with polyarteritis nodosa need combination therapy. Thus, in these disorders, experience with the underlying disease enables the physician to determine when to use another agent such as cyclophosphamide.

The dosage, route, and duration of corticosteroid therapy may also vary with the underlying disease. Having a clear idea of the goal of treatment, features to monitor, and the end point of therapy is important when instituting prednisone. Some diseases require certain doses; in temporal arteritis prednisone must be initiated at a dosage of $\geq$ 60 mg/day (it may then be slowly tapered to 20–30 mg/day) and treatment must be prolonged (> 12 months) because shorter regimens have resulted in devastating relapses.

In addition to the well-described side effects of acute and chronic corticosteroid therapy, there are specific effects which impact vascular diseases. These include a potential to augment vasoconstriction and platelet aggregation. Corticosteriod treatment of vasculitis may truly create a "double-edged sword" [6].

3 Cyclophosphamide

Cyclophosphamide is an alkylating nitrogen mustard that crosslinks DNA, interfering with cell division and thus preventing clonal expansion of B and T lymphocytes. In addition to cytotoxicity, immunologic effects include suppression of immunoglobulin production, diminished antigen-induced proliferation of helper and effector T cells, and reduced cytotoxicity of macrophages. Early evaluations of cyclophosphamide suggested that acute high doses principally suppressed humoral immunity while chronic doses affected cell-mediated immune mechanisms. More recently, influences of cyclophosphamide on endothelial cells are also being explored.

Cyclophosphamide was effectively added to therapeutic immunosuppressive regimens of systemic necrotizing vasculitis in 1973 [10]. It has dramatically reduced the mortality of Wegener's granulomatosis as well as isolated angiitis of the CNS and polyarteritis nodosa. In other diseases it is a useful adjunct, either to reduce the dosage and side effects of prednisone or for corticosteroid failures. It is most often prescribed either in a daily oral dose or as an intermittent intravenous bolus. Oral cyclophosphamide is usually prescribed at a dose of 1–2 mg/kg per day. Hydration is important to prevent hemorrhagic cystitis and reduce the incidence of bladder malignancies. Monitoring of the white blood cell count for the limiting factor of neutropenia < 1500 is essential in dosage management.

More recently, bolus intravenous cyclophosphamide has been tried with the aim of reducing total dosage and side effects. Different protocols of pulse cyclophosphamide administration have been employed; the dose, total number, and frequency of pulses are often adjusted depending on the patient's response and the development of side effects [8]. Pulse cyclophosphamide has been effective in lupus nephritis [30] and systemic vasculitis [35] but, despite initial improvement, in Wegener's granulomatosis there may a higher relapse rate than with standard cyclophosphamide therapy [17].

Isolated angiitis of the CNS is an unusual disease and randomized controlled studies are not feasible; we must, therefore, rely on series of patients accumulated over the years. When the diagnosis of isolated angiitis of the CNS is firmly established, almost all patients either do not respond to or relapse on high-dose prednisone (> 60 mg/day) alone. Combination cyclophosphamide/prednisone therapy is more effective and has fewer side effects [31].

4 Cyclosporine

Cyclosporine, a cyclic endecapeptide extracted from the fungus *Taiypocladium inflatum* Gams, has dramatically affected the treatment of organ transplantation. Cyclosporine's immune effects are selective; it inhibits production of IL-2 by T lymphocytes [23]. The efficacy of cyclosporine in various autoimmune diseases is under investigation. Together with an adrenergic blocking agent, it minimizes vessel permeability in rats with experimental retinal vasculitis [23]. However, in the rabbit serum sickness model of vasculitis, cyclosporine pretreatment increases multifocal organ damage and hemorrhage, ostensibly because of decreased endothelial cell prostacyclin production [32]. The side effects of nephrotoxicity and hypertension limit its widespread use in human vasculitis, although therapeutic benefit is occasionally reported in patients who are refractory to traditional regimens.

5 Azathioprine

Azathioprine, a purine analogue, inhibits protein and antibody synthesis in vitro. Immunoglobulin G production appears more easily suppressed than that of immunoglobulin M. The timing of drug treatment to antigenic challenge markedly affects the result of antibody production, even in relatively resistant species such as man. The effects on cell-mediated immune mechanisms are both specific and nonspecific, but again blocking of sensitization is most effective. Perhaps it is for these reasons that azathioprine has less immunodepressive activity than other agents. It is most often used in the vasculitides in patients who cannot tolerate cyclophosphamide. Overall it is considered less effective than cyclophosphamide, but controlled studies have not been done and are needed. A recent study reported that azathioprine ameliorated the ocular manifestations of Behçet's disease [38].

6 Methotrexate

Methotrexate is a folic acid analogue that acts by inhibiting dihydrofolate reductase. Cells are depleted of folate, with resulting inhibition of purine synthesis and blockage of DNA formation in animals. In vivo studies in animals and humans show that methotrexate suppresses both cell-mediated and humoral immunity. Despite its demonstrated efficacy in the therapy of rheumatoid arthritis, methotrexate is not established in the treatment of vasculitis. In several patients with isolated angiitis of the CNS, methotrexate did not control relapses.

7 Pheresis (Plasma Exchange and Leukopheresis)

Pheresis, the selective removal of plasma or cellular components from the blood, has a simple rationale. Physically removing from the blood substances that cause a disease should improve a patient's condition. Although it is demonstrably effective in controlled studies of Goodpasture's syndrome, certain hyperviscosity states, thrombotic thrombocytopenic purpura, Guillain-Barré, and myasthenia gravis, its efficacy in connective tissue and vasculitic diseases is unsubstantiated [2]. Pheresis has been used in polyarteritis nodosa, particularly that associated with hepatitis B viremia [14].

Plasma exchanges are able to remove immune complexes and to facilitate physiologic removal of complexes by the reticulendothelial system. In the absence of controlled studies, it is difficult to determine if pheresis improves the morbidity and mortality over the standard treatment with prednisone and cyclophosphamide. Pheresis must be combined with an immunosuppressive regimen to prevent a rebound occurrence of immune complexes. In the cell-mediated vasculitides, pheresis of a series of patients has not been reported. The mechanisms by which it would be effective are problematic.

8 Monoclonal Antibody Therapy

Monoclonal antibodies directed against surface markers on lymphocytes are potentially useful as selective therapeutic agents in a variety of immunologically mediated diseases [21, 28]. Current research utilizes antibodies that may block receptors for antigen, adhesion, or growth factors or may block effector cells (via complement activation or Fc binding). The more specific an antibody is, the less likely it is that there will be compromise of normal immune function.

Anti-T-cell monoclonal antibodies are an effective adjunct therapy in allograft rejection. Anti-CD4 and anti-CD11 monoclonal antibodies are potentially useful in cell-mediated inflammatory disorders. Their immunosuppressive effects are more focused than those of immunosuppressive medications such as cyclophosphamide. A serious side effect is the development of antibodies to the murine molecules, with subsequent immune complex disease. Current techniques in molecular biology should enable the generation of human antibodies from heavy and light chain genes with any required specificity. Depending on the size of the molecules and the deliberate insertion of randomness, these antibodies might be more effective and less immunogenic than murine antibodies. They would then be extremely interesting antibodies to try in the therapy of vasculitis.

Monoclonal antibodies to other molecules such as the IL-2 receptor might also modify recurrent inflammation. IL-2 is produced in response to processed and presented antigen; it interacts with specific IL-2 receptors to induce clonal T-cell proliferation. The balance of T-cell subsets, generation of γ-interferon, and NK cell function are all highly dependent on IL-2 synthesis and IL-2 receptor-driven endocytosis. Antibody directed at the IL-2 receptor would be more narrowly targeted than T-cell depletion.

Monoclonal antibodies, anti-CD4 and campath-1H, have successfully induced a short-term remission in one patient with systemic vasculitis refractory to conventional immunosuppression [34].

9 Intravenous Immunoglobulin

Intravenous immunoglobulin, initially used about 10 years ago for the treatment of primary immunodeficiency disease, effectively supplies anti-infectious agent antibodies by passive immunization [9, 12]. It was incidentally noted at the time to improve thrombocytopenia. Although the exact mechanism of this effect remains unknown, possible explanations include:
1. An effect on the Fc receptor of phagocytic cells and B lymphocytes, reducing their effector functions,
2. Production of anti-idiotypic antibodies, or
3. Prevention of activated complement components from reaching their targets [9]. Despite an occasional scattered report, the utility of intravenous immunoglobulins in the vasculitides is not established.

10 Antiprostaglandin

In the diseased blood vessel, endothelium-dependent smooth muscle relaxation is impaired. Both vasoconstriction and secondary platelet aggregation are increased. The endothelial peptide endothelin is a smooth muscle contractor, and increased levels of endothelin are present in some diseases. Anti-inflammatory and antivasospastic effects of prostaglandin E1 infusion have been reported [16]. The size of the vessel involved appears to be a limiting factor. There would be minimal effect of prostaglandin E_1 infusion in peripheral neuropathy due to vasa nervorum infarction and other small vessels too small to contain muscle cells. Side effects are unusual but noteworthy. The vasodilatory effect could result in hypotension (potentially serious in patients with ischemic bowel) and steal syndromes.

11 Antiplatelet Agents And Anticoagulation

In certain of the vasculitides, there is evidence of a coagulopathy. Active Takayasu's disease is associated with hyperfibrinogenemia and hypofibrinolytic activity. Studies in patients with Kawasaki's disease reveal thrombocytosis, diminished fibrinolytic activity, and increased platelet-derived β-thromboglobulin. Fewer data exist for other vasculitides, but thrombosis is a common clinical and histologic feature. Practically, glucocorticoid therapy inhibits endothelial production of prostacyclin but has little effect on platelet thromboxane. Thus, although corticosteroids reduce the inflammation in the infiltrate in the vessel wall, platelet activation, thrombus deposition, and vasoconstriction continue. A potentially simple solution with minimal side effects would be to continue low-dose aspirin during immunosuppressive therapy. This has not been rigorously studied.

Anticoagulation with heparin or coumadin therapy, although theoretically useful, has practical limitations. Many of the vasculitides demonstrate histologic evidence of perivascular hemorrhage. The risk of intracranial hemorrhage in patients treated with anticoagulation is potentially high.

12 Colchicine

Colchicine is a potent anti-inflammatory and immunosuppressant medication which also blocks axonal transport. It effectively suppresses phagocytic function of granulocytes and macrophages. Additionally, enhancement of antibody production and suppression of T-cell subsets have been demonstrated. Despite its use as a remedy for over 200 years in gout, its mechanism of action in this disorder has never been clarified. Several studies suggest it may be useful in Behçet's disease.

Table 1. Standard regimens for treatment of vasculitis

Disease	Agent(s) of choice	Other agents	Selected references
Polyarteritis nodosa	Prednisone/ cyclophosphamide	Prednisone alone	13, 14, 31
Hypersensitivity vasculitis	Remove inciting agent	Prednisone, dapsone	25, 31
Wegener's granulomatosis	Prednisone/ cyclophosphamide	Cotrimoxazol (limited WG)	7, 17, 18, 26, 33
Lymphomatoid granulomatosis	?		11, 32
Temporal arteritis	Prednisone		3, 20, 25
Takayasu's disease	Prednisone	Prednisone, cyclophosphamide	15, 24, 27, 36
Isolated angiitis of CNS	Prednisone/ cyclophosphamide		1, 31, 37
Behçet's disease	?	Prednisone colchicine, azathioprine, cyclophosphamide	38

13 Dapsone

Dapsone appears to suppress myleperoxidase H_2O_2- and halide-mediated cytotoxicity in polymorphonuclear leukocytes. Thus dapsone should be and is most effective in leukocyoclastic vasculitis which contains a prominent polymorphonuclear cell infiltrate [19]. Its efficacy in dermatitis herpetiformis and erythema elevatum diutinum was established in the 1950s. It has some use in vasculitis complicating rheumatoid arthritis, probably because of the role of polymorphonuclear cells in immune complex-mediated vasculitis. Its variable efficacy in the visceral manifestations, relegate this therapy to cases where other therapy fails. Benefit in the cell-mediated vasculitides cannot be anticipated. Some small studies did not show a benefit of dapsone therapy in temporal arteritis.

14 Conclusion

Treatment of patients with vasculitis requires expertise with a spectrum of vasculitides and autoimmune diseases in order to appreciate the potential for overlap syndromes or evolution of a specific diagnosis over time. Experience in the use of immunosuppressant medications is also important because of the wide range of potential and actual side effects. Side effects can occur with any of these agents, and the physician should be thoroughly acquainted with all potential side effects before initiating treatment. Most patients do well on the standard regimens shown in Table 1. More difficult are those patients who only partially respond to treatment. The physician must determine whether the clinical effects are due to persistent inflammation or other causes. Excluding infection should remain a high priority. Ischemia may result not only from the inflammation but also from thrombosis and/or hemorrhage.

References

1. Budzilovich GN, Feigin I, Siegel H (1963) Granulomatous angiitis of the nervous system. Arch Pathol 76:250–256
2. Campion EW (1992) Desperate diseases and plasmapheresis. N Engl J Med 326(21):1425–1427
3. Caselli RJ, Hunder GG, Whisnant JP (1988) Neurologic disease in biopsy-proven giant cell (temporal) arteritis. Neurology 38:352–359
4. Clements PJ, Davis J (1986) Cytotoxic drugs: their clinical applications to the rheumatic diseases. Semin Arthritis Rheum 15(4):231–254
5. Conn DL (1989) Subspeciality clinics: Rheumatology. Update on systemic necrotizing vasculitis. Mayo Clin Proc 64:535–543
6. Conn DL, Tompkins RB, Nichols WL (1988) Glucocorticoids in the management of vasculitis – a double edge sword? J Rheumatol 15:1181–1183
7. DeRemee RA (1988) The treatment of Wegener's granulomatosis with trimethoprim-/sulfamethoxazole: illusion or vision? Arthritis Rheum 31(8):1068–1072
8. De Vita SD, Bombardieri S (1991) Cyclophosphamide pulses in the treatment of rheumatic diseases: an update. Clin Exp Rheumatol 9:179–193
9. Dietrich G, Kaveri SV, Kazatchkine MD (1992) Modulation of autoimmunity by intravenous immune globulin through interaction with the function of the immune/idiotypic network. Clin Immunol Immunopathol 62:S73-S81
10. Fauci AS, Wolff SM (1973) Wegener's granulomatosis: studies in eighteen patients and a review of the literature. Medicine 52:535–561
11. Fauci AS, Haynes BF, Costa J, Katz P, Wolff SM (1982) Lymphomatoid granulomatosis. Prospective clinical and therapeutic experience over 10 years. N Engl J Med 306:68–74
12. Frank MM, Basta M, Fries LF (1992) The effects of intravenous immune globulin on complement-dependent immune damage of cells and tissues. Clin Immunol Immunopathol 62:982–986
13. Giulian D, Woodward J, Young DG, Krebs JF, Lachman LB Interleukin-1 injected into mamalian brain stimulates astrogliosis and neovascularization. J Neurosci 8:2485–2490 1988
14. Guillevin L, Jarrousse B, Lok C, et al (1991) Longterm followup after treatment of polyarteritis nodosa and Churg–Strass angiitis with comparison of steroids, plasma exchange and cyclophosphamide to steroids and plasma exchange. A prospective randomized trial of 71 patients. J Rheumatol 18:567–574
15. Hall S, Barr W, Lie JT, Stanson AW, Kazmier FJ, Hunder GG (1985) Takayasu arteritis. A study of 32 North American patients. Medicine 64(2):89–99
16. Hauptman HW, Ruddy S, Roberts WN (1991) Reversal of the vasospastic component of lupus vasculopathy by infusion of prostaglandin E1. J Rheumatol 18:1747–1752
17. Hoffman GS, Kerr GS, Leavitt RY, et al (1992) Wegener's granulomatosis: an analysis of 158 patients. Ann Int Med 116(6):488–498
18. Hoffman GS, Leavitt RY, Fleisher TA, Minor JR, Fauci AS (1990) Treatment of Wegener's granulomatosis with intermittent high-dose intravenous cyclophosphamide. Am J Med 89(4):403–410

19. Holtman JH, Neustadt DH, Klein J, Callen JP (1990) Dapsone is an effective therapy for the skin lesions of subacute cutaneous lupus erythematosus and urticarial vasculitis in a patient with C2 deficiency. J Rheumatol 17(9):1222–1225
20. Hunder GG, Sheps SG, Allen GL, Joyce JW (1975) Daily and alternate-day corticosteroid regimes in treatment of giant cell arteritis. Comparison in a prospective study. Ann Int Med 82:613–618
21. Isaacs JD, Clark MR, Greenwood J, Waldmann H (1992) Therapy with monoclonal antibodies. J Immunol 148:3062–3071
22. Jesus AD, Talal N (1990) Practical use of immunosuprressive drugs in autoimmune rheumatic diseases. Crit Care Med 18:S132-S137
23. Kahan BD (1989) Drug therapy. Cyclosporine. N Engl J Med 321:1725–1736
24. Kanaide H, Takeshita A, Nakamura M (1982) Etiologic aspects of coagulopathy in Takayasu's aortitis. Am Heart J 104:1039–1045
25. Kissel JT, Rammohan KW (1991) Pathogenesis and therapy of nervous system vasculitis. Clin Neuropharmacol 14:28–48
26. Leavitt RY, Hoffman GS, Fauci AS (1988) The role of trimethoprim/sulfamethoxazole in the treatment of Wegener's granulomatosis. Arthritis Rheum 31:1073–1074
27. Mason WH, Jordan SC, Saki R, Takahashi M, Berstein B (1985) Circulating immune complexes in Kawasaki syndrome. Pediatr Infect Dis J 4:48
28. Mathieson PW, Cobbold SP, Hale G, et al (1990) Monoclonal-antibody therapy in systemic vasculitis. N Engl J Med 323:250–254
29. Mathieu A, Carcassi U (1989) Cytotoxic drugs in systemic autoimmune diseases. Clin Exp Rheumatol 7/S3:181–186
30. McCune WJ, Golbus J, Zeldes W, Bohlke P, Dunne R, Fox DA (1988) Clinical and immunologic effects of monthly administration of intravenous cyclophosphamide in severe systemic lupus erythematosus. N Engl J Med 318:1423–1431
31. Moore PM, Fauci AS (1981) Neurologic manifestations of systemic vasculitis. A retrospective and prospective study of the clinicopathologic features and responses to therapy in 25 patients. Am J Med 71:517–524
32. Neild GH, Ivory K, Williams DG (1984) Severe systemic vascular necrosis in cyclosporin-treatment rabbits with acute serum sickness. Br J Exp Pathol 65:731–743
33. Patton WF, Lynch JP(1982) Lymphomatoid granulomatosis. Clinicopathologic study of four cases and literature review. Medicine 61:1–12
34. Pirofsky B, Kinzey DM (1992) Intravenous immune globulins. A review of their uses in selected immunodeficiency and autoimmune diseases. Drugs 43:6–14
35. Scott DGI, Bacon PA (1984) Intravenous cyclophosphamide plus methylprednisolone in treatment of systemic rheumatoid vasculitis. Am J Med 76:377–384
36. Shelhamer JH, Voldman DJ, Parrillo JE, Lawley TJ, Johnston MR, Fauci AS (1985) Takayasu's arteritis and its therapy. Ann Int Med 103:121–126
37. Vincent FM (1977) Granulomatous angiitis. N Engl J Med 296:452
38. Yazici H, Pazarli H, Barnes CG, et al (1990) A controlled trial of azathioprine in Behçet's syndrome. N Engl J Med 322:281–285

Subject Index